The Uncomplicated Guide to Diabetes Complications

D0484534

Edited by
Marvin E. Levin, MD and
Michael A. Pfeifer, MD

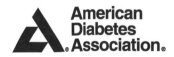
American
Diabetes
Association.

Book Acquisitions	Robert J. Anthony
Editors	Sherrye Landrum and Aime M. Ballard
Production Director	Carolyn R. Segree
Production Coordinator	Peggy M. Rote
Desktop Publishing	Harlowe Typography, Inc.
Design	Wickham & Associates, Inc.
Illustrations	Duckwall Productions

Printed in Canada
1 3 5 7 9 10 8 6 4 2

American Diabetes Association
1660 Duke Street
Alexandria, Virginia 22314

Library of Congress Cataloging-in-Publication Data
The uncomplicated guide to diabetes complications / edited by Marvin
   E. Levin and Michael A. Pfeifer.
      p.   cm.
   Includes bibliographical references and index.
   ISBN 0-945448-87-2
   1. Diabetes—Complications—Popular works.   I. Levin, Marvin E.,
   1924–   .   II. Pfeifer, Michael A.
   RC660.4.U53   1998
   616.4'62—dc21   98-7166
                                   CIP

Books Editorial Advisory Board

Table of Contents

Introduction

Two miracles, the discoveries of insulin and antibiotics, have significantly prolonged the life of people with diabetes. That is the good news. The bad news is that longer life spans allow many people with diabetes to develop complications of the disease.

Diabetic complications can be prevented and treated. This requires the expertise of many medical specialties, so to help you, we have gathered in this book the knowledge and contributions of many world-renowned specialists. The complications that commonly occur in diabetes include eye disease, now the leading cause of blindness in the U.S.; atherosclerosis, hardening of the arteries, which can lead to heart attack and stroke; loss of nerve function, particularly in the lower extremities, which can lead to painless trauma, ulcerated infection, gangrene, and amputation; and kidney disease, now the leading reason for dialysis. Other diabetic complications include those of the digestive system, impotence, female sexual disorders, dental and skin abnormalities, and psychological disorders.

The complications of diabetes can be prevented or greatly reduced. In addition to improved quality of life, this would result in saving billions of dollars a year in

Medicare costs. The means to this desirable end are to maintain good blood glucose control and to get the following checked regularly:

1. LDL cholesterol
2. Blood pressure
3. Urinary protein
4. Glycated hemoglobin
5. Dilated eye examination
6. Monofilament testing

To further improve your chances of not having a complication, you should stop smoking and get patient education (including meal planning). If you wait until symptoms occur, it will be too late. Any of the six tests above can give abnormal results before you have symptoms, and that is the time to treat them. It is important to get these tests for yourself.

The book deals with how to prevent these complications and, if problems occur, how they can and should be treated. It also points out many of the things your doctor and other health care providers should be doing to prevent and treat complications. All of these treatments should be discussed with and prescribed by your doctors. Never use them without medical supervision or assistance.

As you read the book, you will see that the bottom line—and there is always a bottom line—is repeated over and over: **The most important thing you can do to help prevent complications is to achieve good blood glucose control.**

If you follow the instructions in these chapters, you will have a healthier life, with fewer complications of diabetes.

List of Contributors

Lloyd Paul Aiello, MD, PhD
Paul D. Baker
Jeffrey L. Barnett, MD
Jose Biller, MD, FACP
Michael Camilleri, MD
Culley C. Carson, MD
Jerry D. Cavallerano, OD, PhD
Samuel Dagogo-Jack, MD, FACP
Eva L. Feldman, MD, PhD
Eli A. Friedman, MD
Robert G. Frykberg, DPM, MPH
Martha M. Funnel, MS, RN, CDE
Edward M. Geltman, MD
Saul M. Genuth, MD
Gary W. Gibbons, MD
M. Gilbert Grand, MD
Douglas A. Greene, MD
Mami A. Iwamoto, MD
Sheilah A. Janus
Lois Jovanovic, MD
Jeffrey A. Levin, DMD
Benjamin A. Lipsky, MD

Betsy B. Love, MD
Dordaneh Maleki, MD
Roger Marzano, CPO, Cped
Mark E. Molitch, MD
Mark Peyrot, PhD
Luarinda M. Poirier, RN, MPH, CDE
Venkatraman Rajkumar, MD
Richard R. Rubin, PhD, CDE
Lee J. Sanders, DPM
Leslie R. Schover, PhD
Patricia Schreiner-Engel, PhD
R. Gary Sibbald, MD
James R. Sowers, MD
Ilana P. Spector, PhD
Mark A. Sperling, MD
Martin J. Stevens, MD
David E.R. Sutherland, MD, PhD
Aruna Venkatesh, MD
Aaron Vinik, MD, PhD, FCP, FACP
Katherine V. Williams, MD
Rena R. Wing, PhD

1

Acute Complications

Case study

MJ is 47 years old and has had type 1 diabetes for 20 years. She is suffering from an intestinal flu with vomiting and hasn't eaten in 24 hours. Because she hasn't eaten, she has mistakenly decided not to take any insulin. Now she feels really awful, dizzy, and short of breath. The vomiting continues. She calls her health care provider, who suspects diabetic ketoacidosis (DKA) and tells her to go to the emergency room immediately.

Case study

LP is 72 years old, lives alone, and was just diagnosed with type 2 diabetes last week. He has been taking prednisone, a steroid, for 4 weeks for another serious condition. Now he is extremely thirsty and urinating often. He feels exhausted. Sensing that something is wrong, he goes to see his physician and finds that his blood pressure is low and his blood glucose level is 925 mg/dl. By now he is sleepy and lethargic. He is experiencing hyperglycemic hyperosmolar nonketotic coma (HHNC).

Case study

PJ is 17 years old and has had type 1 diabetes for 5 years. She is learning that she can eat whatever she wants but still not gain weight if she lets her blood sugars stay way above normal. She goes to a slumber party and stays up all night, eating pizza but not injecting any insulin. When she arrives home, she is thirsty, lethargic, and nauseated. Her mother thinks it may be DKA and takes her to the emergency room.

Introduction

Diabetes is a chronic, lifetime disease. All patients can learn to balance and maintain blood glucose control through daily treatment with healthy eating, exercise, and medication if needed. Keeping blood glucose close to normal frees you from day-to-day symptoms of high blood glucose levels and wards off the later complications that affect eyes, kidneys, and nerves. There are, however, acute complications of diabetes that can cause sudden, serious, and even life-threatening events. They either are preventable, for the most part, or can be treated before hospitalization is required or any damage is done. This chapter describes the biochemical background, causes, symptoms, treatment, and preventive measures for the two major acute complications: 1) DKA, also sometimes called diabetic acidosis or diabetic coma, and 2) HHNC.

In the latest complete data available (1989–1991), approximately 100,000 people of all ages, with most being less than 45, had been hospitalized for DKA. In contrast, there were approximately 11,000 hospitalizations for HHNC, with the vast majority being older than 65. Of every 1,000 people with diabetes, 2–5 may suffer DKA in any given year. These are disturbing numbers, indeed.

What is DKA?

The disturbance in handling glucose or carbohydrates is not the only thing wrong in diabetes. Fats and proteins are also profoundly disturbed when insulin is lacking or ineffective. The term *metabolism* includes all of the chemical reactions the body performs to transform food into the energy and structures that support life. DKA is a metabolic disturbance in which blood glucose levels rise too high and the body becomes very dehydrated and begins to burn excessive amounts of fat for energy. This in turn causes the body to produce ketones, a product of burning fat. In this situation, the body also produces excess acid. The products, excess ketones and acids, give this condition the name ketoacidosis. Such a disturbance can be life-threatening.

What causes DKA?

When you don't have enough insulin or it's not working right, glucose cannot get from your bloodstream into insulin's target cells, especially muscle cells and fat cells. The glucose cannot be oxidized for energy without insulin. Without insulin, excess glucose is formed from protein (amino acids) in the liver cells and flows into the blood. In DKA, both factors—slower exit of glucose from the blood and faster entrance of glucose into the blood—raise glucose levels in the blood. Exactly how high they can go depends on still another organ, the kidney.

The role of the kidney is more complicated to explain (Figure 1-1). The kidney saves glucose, because the glucose molecule is essential to so many body functions. Normally, glucose is filtered out of the blood in one part of the kidney, and returned to the blood in another part. However, when blood glucose levels rise above 180 mg/dl, the kidney lets the excess glucose be excreted in the urine.

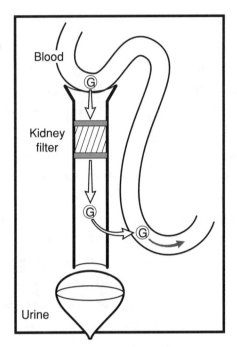

Normal
Blood Glucose
100 mg/dl

Blood

Kidney
filter

Urine

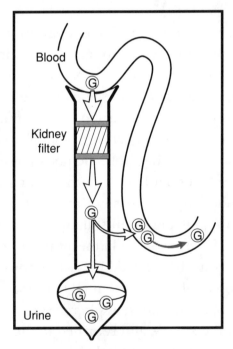

Diabetic
Blood Glucose
200 mg/dl

Blood

Kidney
filter

Urine

Figure 1-1. When blood glucose goes above a certain level, the kidney releases glucose in the urine.

This is how the kidney helps keep blood glucose from going even higher above the normal range than it already has.

The glucose must be dissolved in water to be excreted. So, your body needs more water. That is why two of the symptoms of uncontrolled diabetes are extreme thirst and excessive urination. Finally, however, the kidney excretes more fluid than you drink and your body becomes severely dehydrated so that the kidney cannot filter much glucose out of the blood. Your blood glucose can rise to levels of 400–1,000 mg/dl (and, although rarely, sometimes higher).

The glucose excreted in urine takes with it huge amounts of water and sodium chloride (salt). Sodium chloride is responsible for keeping enough water in the bloodstream so that the blood pumped by the heart can carry sufficient oxygen and nutrients to every cell in the body. As more and more water and sodium chloride are lost in the urine, the volume of blood shrinks and circulation of the blood is reduced. You become dried out (dehydrated), limiting what the kidney can do. The reduced kidney function contributes further to raising your blood glucose, and a vicious cycle begins. Other key substances such as potassium, phosphate, and magnesium and the nitrogen from the amino acid building blocks of protein are also lost in the urine, with potentially dangerous consequences for the function of your heart and other organs.

What does ketoacidosis mean?

Ordinarily, the body burns fat and carbohydrates to get carbon dioxide and water. To keep this process going efficiently, some glucose must be added to the fuel mix, which requires insulin. When insulin either is unavailable or doesn't work properly, two things happen. First, fat is released from storage cells and broken down for use as an energy source (ketoacids and acetone are byproducts of this breakdown of fat). Then, the high fat levels in the blood flood the liver and exceed its capacity to burn the fat completely. The process is hampered because fat cells and liver cells aren't able to use the glucose that is in the blood. The result is that fat is not completely burned but stops at a chemical half-way point—ketoacids or ketone bodies—before carbon dioxide and water are formed (Figure 1-2). The ketoacids are made in huge quantities, and they pile up in blood after they are released from the liver. The two ketoacids—acetoacetic acid and beta-hydroxybutyric acid—are the *keto* in ketoacidosis. They also are excreted in your urine where acetoacetic acid and another byproduct called acetone can be detected by Ketotest or Ketostix.

Now, what about *acidosis*? The two ketoacids are relatively strong acids. Think of them like acetic acid in vinegar. The body cannot tolerate ketoacids for long. They must be neutralized, and the process that the body uses is to convert them to carbon dioxide, which is exhaled by the lungs. People with DKA must breathe more rapidly and deeply. Acetone is exhaled, in part, through the lungs. This causes the breath to have a fruity odor. If the lungs did not get rid of the extra carbon dioxide, the high acid level of the blood would poison all the body cells, and life would cease. That's why insulin was truly a magical life-saving drug in the first few years of its use—and it still is.

What does protein have to do with DKA?

Proteins can be considered the most important molecules in the body next to DNA molecules (genes). The walls of cells, the other structural parts of cells, the muscle fibers that give us movement, the tendons, the bones, and the enzymes—the chemical wizards that catalyze millions of reactions every minute—all these and many more are made up of protein molecules. Surprisingly for such essen-

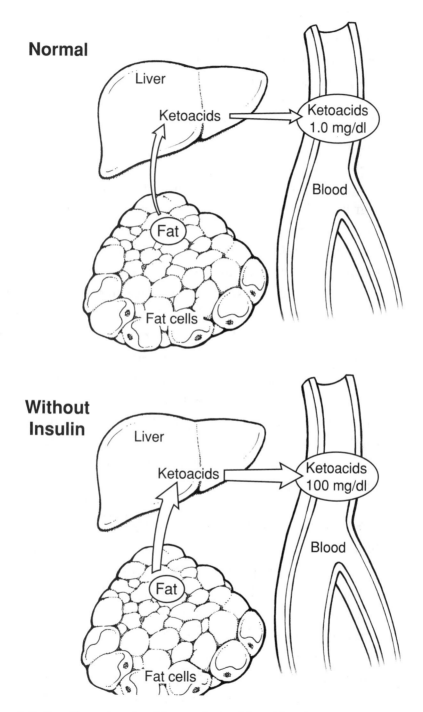

Figure 1-2. Ketoacids are a byproduct of the incomplete breakdown of fat in the liver.

tial molecules, proteins are rather fragile. They are constantly being destroyed and therefore have to be rebuilt constantly. Both their destruction and their resynthesis are regulated by insulin. Without insulin, breakdown of proteins speeds up and the rebuilding process slows. Your body loses proteins as amino acids and other nitrogen-containing chemicals in the urine. The cells literally start to melt away in DKA. The potassium, phosphate, and magnesium in the cells are lost with the proteins and are dragged out into the urine along with glucose. Old photographs of people with type 1 diabetes at this stage show them to be as emaciated as concentration camp victims. Of course, these days, the short time an individual is in DKA before receiving treatment does not allow such huge losses of body proteins; however, the process has certainly begun. To add to the problems in DKA, the broken-down protein is also changed into glucose and ketoacids and contributes to the rising blood glucose levels and degree of acidosis.

To summarize, the severe abnormalities in full-blown DKA are high blood glucose levels, accumulation of acid in the blood and cells, marked loss of salt and water from the body, and ongoing destruction of body protein with loss of amino acids as nitrogen along with potassium, phosphate, and magnesium in the urine.

What puts you at risk for developing DKA?

Not having enough insulin puts you at risk for DKA. Most cases occur in people with type 1 diabetes—the type of diabetes that usually develops in younger patients. In one-tenth to one-fifth of all instances, the individuals did not even know they had diabetes—for example, school-age children sent off to camp, where neither they nor their counselors recognize that frequent urination or bed-wetting are signs of diabetes. Most people with undiagnosed diabetes have suffered from frequent urination, thirst, loss of weight, and blurred vision for 4–8 weeks before they come to the hospital or physician.

People who know that they have type 1 diabetes but have an interruption in their insulin schedule also get DKA. The time between stopping insulin and going into DKA varies a great deal. The quickest example occurs in patients who use insulin infusion pumps. If the catheter gets blocked or the pump stops delivering insulin for any reason, DKA can occur within 6–12 hours, because all the insulin used in the pump is regular or Humalog (lispro) insulin, both of which disappear rapidly from the body. (Note: This is not a reason to avoid the insulin pump, which may have advantages for some patients.) In contrast, DKA may take several days to develop after stopping NPH, lente, or ultralente insulin, because these insulins hang around longer in the skin. The more years a person has had type 1 diabetes, the quicker DKA is likely to develop when treatment is interrupted, because there are no beta cells left to provide even the small amount of insulin it takes to prevent this condition.

Even if you take all prescribed insulin doses, DKA can occur. This is usually brought about by another medical illness—an infection such as strep throat or intestinal flu. The latter is especially bad because it produces vomiting and/or diarrhea, both of which decrease body fluids and make dehydration worse. The stress of an illness or surgery causes your body to release hormones, including cortisone, glucagon, epinephrine, and growth hormone. Each of these opposes insulin action in its own way. Together, they raise blood glucose and ketoacid levels. In type 1 patients who have little or no insulin reserve, DKA can develop quickly unless extra insulin is given. Patients with type 2 diabetes can develop DKA even though they have insulin. In this situation, we say they have insulin resistance, that is, resistance to the action of insulin, and therefore need additional insulin to correct the elevated blood glucose and DKA.

Commonly, as in the first case presented in this chapter, people cause DKA by not taking insulin if they are vomiting or have diarrhea. They make the mistake of thinking that because they are not eating, their blood glucose will be low. They forget that with type 1 diabetes, your body doesn't make insulin. So if you don't inject insulin, your blood glucose will rise even if you haven't eaten.

On rare occasions, no illness can be found, but DKA still occurs. In some of these instances, we believe the stress causing DKA may be emotional, such as a distressing school, work, family, or social situation. Or the cause may be an internal crisis of which you are not aware. Emotional upsets can cause repeated episodes of DKA only weeks or months apart, and a persistent emotional crisis can remain undetected unless your physician or family is persistent about helping you unveil the problem to yourself. You may need to resolve it with professional help.

These uncommon situations are particularly likely to occur in adolescents, who are trying to deal with the physical, psychological, and social changes of puberty in addition to diabetes. The problem is especially dangerous when it leads teenagers to stop taking insulin surreptitiously as a means of testing themselves, their diabetes, and their family's love and attention. Teenage girls will sometimes keep themselves in poor glucose control to stay slender. They have discovered that by allowing themselves to have higher-than-normal glucose levels, they can eat whatever they want and not gain weight. The problem is that it takes very little to send them into ketoacidosis. These girls are seen multiple times a year in the emergency room in DKA. If the situation is recognized, then some compromise can be reached to ensure them better metabolic balance and better health.

Can people with type 2 diabetes develop DKA?

Yes, DKA can occur in older people with type 2 diabetes. It is brought on by major medical illness such as a heart attack, trauma such as a hip fracture, or an emergency surgical condition such as appendicitis. Whenever there is no obvious cause for DKA, your physician must look for unusual infections that may be masked by the DKA itself. These include meningitis, serious external ear infections, fungal infections in the nose, dental infections, and even rectal abscesses. Finally, adrenal or pituitary glands may secrete excess amounts of the counterinsulin hormones mentioned above. In rare cases, this may present as DKA. You might say that while DKA itself is easy to recognize, identifying its cause may take detective work by you and your diabetes care team.

What are the symptoms of DKA?

With few exceptions, you feel awful. The rising blood glucose levels have caused frequent urination and extreme thirst. The resulting dehydration causes a parched tongue, weakness, and dizziness on standing. The high blood-acid level causes nausea, vomiting, and, rarely, abdominal pain so severe that it mimics diseases such as appendicitis. Diarrhea is not a symptom of DKA, and its presence may point to gastroenteritis as the illness causing DKA. You hyperventilate to "blow off" all the carbon dioxide being formed from neutralizing the acid in the blood. This often gives you the sensation of being short of breath, and to the observer, it looks like "air hunger." After many hours of high blood glucose levels, the brain cells also become dehydrated and function abnormally. Lethargy, sleepiness, and confusion result and can eventually end up as coma, with you being unresponsive to anything but pain. Although a complete recovery is still possible from coma, time is of the essence in getting you to a hospital and beginning treatment. Fortunately, complete coma from DKA is becoming increasingly rare in the United States.

How is DKA treated?

The most pressing need is to give intravenous water and salt. This is done rapidly in the first 1–2 hours of treatment to restore circulation to all the body tissues. This also improves blood flow to the kidneys and allows those organs to remove glucose from the blood more efficiently (Figure 1-2). More intravenous fluid is then given slowly over the next 8–24 hours until all the body water losses have been made up. This may require as much as 5–10 quarts or liters of fluid. Although intravenous fluids alone cannot reverse DKA, they can slightly lower blood glucose by allowing the kidneys to filter more glucose and excrete it in the urine.

The next need is to supply the missing insulin. This is also done intravenously whenever possible to guarantee a quick and reliable effect. Besides bringing blood glucose down to a more reasonable range (150–250 mg/dl), the insulin stops the release and the burning of so much fat. In turn, this stops the production of the ketoacids and gradually corrects the state of acidosis.

Insulin also stops the breakdown of protein and stimulates the return of amino acids, potassium, phosphate, and magnesium into the cells where the protein stores can be rebuilt. It is critical always to give sufficient potassium with the insulin. Otherwise, the potassium may fall to dangerously low levels in the blood because the cells soak it up so quickly. A very low blood potassium level can interfere with the action of the heart. Therefore, the physician follows not only glucose but also potassium blood levels. Replacing potassium appropriately can be critical. Occasionally, phosphate is given. The rarest are circumstances where magnesium falls to critically low levels in the blood and causes heart irregularities that require emergency treatment with intravenous magnesium.

The acidosis is corrected by insulin treatment alone. Occasionally, however, the level of acid is so high in the blood that the acid itself is endangering you. In those instances, a sterile liquid form of baking soda is given intravenously to neutralize the dangerous excess of acid and allow time for insulin to stop the production of more acid. Appropriate antibiotics are given for any bacterial infection.

Because the various components of DKA treatment must be coordinated, you should be closely monitored by nurses and physicians. Your pulse, blood pressure, and mental status are checked hourly, and temperature less often. Blood samples for measurement of glucose, acid levels, potassium, and phosphate are taken frequently. To prevent vomiting, no fluids are allowed by mouth. All intravenous fluids given and all urine passed must be accurately measured and charted to be sure that you are actually regaining body fluids. Electrocardiograms (ECGs) are performed. It is small wonder that most patients get very little rest during such activity and are often very tired and somewhat cranky the next day.

By the next day, things are usually squared away, and the intravenous insulin can be stopped. If all is well, your usual insulin program is restarted or a new program is begun as appropriate. If nausea is gone, you can begin to eat (often between yawns). If no serious infection or other complications are found, discharge from the hospital is usually accomplished after 2–3 days of reestablishing daily glucose control. At the same time, you and your family are educated about DKA and how to prevent it.

How can you prevent DKA?

It is certainly far better for you—and easier for everyone concerned—to prevent DKA or stop it in its earliest stage than to enter the hospital in a coma. Prevention begins with knowing when to be concerned about the possibility of DKA and how to test for its presence. This is the reason for so-called sick-day management. Any illness, even the common cold, should trigger you and your family's early warning system. Fever, nausea, and vomiting even one time are danger flags that call for immediate assessment of your metabolic status.

If you have any of these symptoms, blood glucose and urine ketone tests should be done immediately. If the blood glucose level is less than 250 mg/dl and urine ketones are negative, only take your usual insulin doses and continue to monitor blood glucose and urine ketones every 4 hours until the illness has passed. Drink fluids of all kinds in generous amounts. If you vomit a second time, your blood glucose increases to more than 250 mg/dl, or the urine test for ketones becomes positive, call your health care provider at once for advice.

You must pay attention to vomiting that limits or prevents fluid intake, because it greatly increases your risk of dehydration. If the illness is gastroenteritis, diarrhea may add to the loss of fluids and salts. Infants and young children are particularly vulnerable to DKA because they normally begin with less fluid in their body, and the elderly have less kidney function to begin with. Replacement of lost water and salt can be accomplished with bouillon (one standard cube in 8 ounces of water approximates the body's ratio of salt to water). Gatorade or similar products or a solution of glucose, salt, baking soda, and potassium recommended by the World Health Organization usually works as well. Small amounts of fluid taken frequently, for example, 3 ounces every 30 minutes for an adult, are better for you than large amounts drunk rapidly. If blood glucose is running below normal, high carbohydrate fluids, such as fruit juices, regular sodas, or tea with sugar, should be alternated with fluids that contain salt, such as bouillon.

Some physicians provide you with prescriptions in advance for medications for nausea and vomiting such as rectal suppositories and instructions on how to use them. Other physicians want to do this only after being notified that a problem exists or is brewing. Either way, stopping the vomiting is of great importance in preventing DKA because it reduces the risk of dehydration.

The other major principle of prevention is never to stop your insulin injections because of loss of appetite, nausea, vomiting, or fear of hypoglycemia. You may need to change your insulin dose. But there are no dosage rules that always apply to each patient and each situation. That is why frequent testing of blood glucose and urine ketones is essential to navigating through this dangerous period, especially if the first signs of DKA are already present. You may need to test every 2 hours or even in the middle of the night, and communicate the results promptly to your diabetes caregivers. They should give you specific instructions about doses of insulin to be taken each time, and they may give instructions for future doses, depending on later blood glucose and urine ketone test results.

Don't call the doctor without being able to provide up-to-the-minute blood glucose and urine ketone results and an estimate of how much and what kind of fluids you have drunk. If you, your family, physician, and diabetes nurse work together as a true health care team, the risk of DKA caused by 24- to 48-hour viral flu or gastroenteritis can be eliminated. If the infection is bacterial, for example strep throat, antibiotics may speed your recovery, so get prescriptions filled immediately. Once your blood glucose has been kept in a safe range (100–200 mg/dl) for a few hours and ketones have disappeared from your urine, the danger of DKA is generally over.

What are the signs that DKA is getting worse?

Symptoms of DKA may worsen because stress hormones block the usual effects of insulin so that increasingly larger doses are required. Signs that home treatment has not been adequate include continued vomiting, complaints of shortness of breath, and excessive sleepiness. The physician may note breathlessness and a dulling of mental processes by listening to you on the telephone. That's why the physician should communicate directly with you and not a family member. If these symptoms appear, you will need to go to the emergency room, preferably of a hospital used by both you and your physician, for additional help. More sophisticated blood tests measuring the amount of acid in the blood can determine whether DKA has occurred. You can be given fluids and insulin intravenously with salt, glucose, and potassium. The responsibility for management can be shifted from an ill and often tired you or your family to professionals. This treatment can often stop or reverse DKA within 6–12 hours in an emergency room or in a hospital observation unit, and a 2- to 3-day hospital stay can be avoided. The decision of whether to treat at home, directly in the emergency room, or by admission to the hospital is best made by a physician who knows you and your family and home circumstances.

What is hyperglycemic hyperosmolar nonketotic coma (HHNC)?

Many of the things already said about DKA apply equally well to HHNC. *Hyperglycemic* (the first H) means that blood glucose levels are too high. HHNC has a higher average blood glucose (900 mg/dl or higher) than DKA. The blood glucose can climb higher for several reasons. HHNC develops more slowly and gradually. The thirsty patient seems to prefer sweet liquids with higher carbohydrate content. The function of the kidneys is more greatly reduced because the patient becomes more dehydrated. And the patient or caregivers ignore or mistake the symptoms for something else and wait too long to get assistance from the health care team. By the time they do, the loss of salt and especially of plain water from the body can be enormous.

The second H stands for *hyperosmolar* and is a technical way of saying that all of the chemicals contained in blood are now dissolved in much less water. Because of this, water is drawn into the blood from the body cells so that the whole patient is hyperosmolar and very dehydrated. The blood may become so thick that it clots easily, which can cause secondary strokes and heart attacks.

N stands for *nonketotic*. This means that the ketoacids produced in DKA are not produced in large amounts in HHNC and do not build up in the blood to any great degree. The main reason is thought to be that these patients typically have type 2 and not type 1 diabetes. They can still secrete the small amount of insulin it takes to prevent the excessive breakdown of fat and the conversion of fat to ketoacids in the liver (Figure 1-2). Whatever the reason, the lack of high acid levels in the blood actually contributes to the long delay in getting care: you are not alerted by nausea and vomiting that something is very wrong. Similarly, protein is probably not lost to the extent it is in DKA; therefore, losses of amino acids, potassium, phosphate, and magnesium may not be as great.

The C stands for *coma,* a state of unconsciousness that occurs more often in HHNC than in DKA.

Who is at risk of developing HHNC?

Children and young adults almost never get HHNC. The typical patient is an elderly person, who is often living alone or in a nursing home and may be unaware that she or he even has diabetes. A major medical event such as a heart attack or an infection that has spread into the bloodstream from some local site such as the urinary tract or a foot ulcer may start the process. Certain drugs can contribute to a steep rise in blood glucose. Examples are prednisone or other steroids, diuretics such as hydrochlorothiazide, and anticonvulsant medication such as dilantin. Even so, there is usually underlying type 2 diabetes, which needs treatment after the HHNC has been reversed.

What are the symptoms of HHNC?

Some symptoms of HHNC differ from symptoms of DKA. You are usually more dehydrated—literally dried out—with prunelike wrinkled skin. You are more likely to be in shock, that is, to have a very low blood pressure with poor blood flow to many organs and general failure of their vital functions. Most strikingly, coma is much more frequent. Instead of confusion or loss of consciousness, the brain may be so affected by the hyperosmolar state that seizures, paralysis, and other neurological dysfunction can occur. Many patients are initially thought to have had a stroke; yet with complete treatment, the abnormal neurological signs can disappear completely. However, it may take several days for the patient to regain a baseline state of brain function. Despite the lack of acidosis, HHNC is in many ways a more serious acute complication of diabetes than is DKA, and the chances of recovering from it are not as good, even with correct treatment.

What is the treatment for HHNC?

The treatment of HHNC follows the same principles as DKA. Usually only small amounts of insulin are required. The major difference relates to the degree of dehydration and the degree of hyperosmolarity. HHNC patients need emergency fluid flowing to their tissues to get them out of shock and to restore normal blood flow to the heart through the coronary arteries, to the brain, to the kidneys, to the liver and gastrointestinal tract, and to the limbs. Because the elderly patient with type 2 diabetes usually has atherosclerosis with narrowing of the major arteries, improving blood flow and oxygen delivery quickly is vital to prevent complete blockage of one of these major arteries. Such obstructions can cause catastrophic consequences: coronary thrombosis (heart attack), cerebral thrombosis (stroke), a leg artery thrombosis (gangrene and need for amputation), a bowel artery thrombosis (death of a bowel segment and peritonitis), and kidney failure.

Once the blood volume is back to normal, the balance of salt and water in the intravenous fluids must favor water. The intake of fluid and the output of urine must be closely monitored, as must the balance of water, glucose, salt, and indicators of kidney function in the blood. Most HHNC patients remain in a perilous state for several days—much longer than typical DKA patients. Treatment of any infection requiring antibiotics must be aggressive.

How can you prevent HHNC?

You, your family, nursing home personnel, and health care professionals all need to be educated about this condition. Discovery of undetected diabetes by periodic health screening is very important in the vulnerable elderly age group. Close attention to the welfare of elderly relatives who have diabetes coupled with the knowledge presented here can prevent many cases. Likewise, aides and nurses in facilities that care for the aged must be sensitive to the significance of frequent urination or the abrupt appearance of incontinence. Elderly people do not experience thirst as well as younger people do, when the body needs water. Therefore, they and their caregivers need to note how much fluid they drink. Don't write off a decline in mental status as "senile dementia" without being sure that a very high blood glucose level is not the reversible cause. Likewise, don't dismiss a complaint of dizziness, especially on standing, which could signal a low volume of blood, as the result of "hardening of the arteries" in the brain. We need to be as concerned that a person is having a "glucose attack" as we are for heart attacks and the recently coined term *brain attacks*. Nothing is easier or more certain to help a patient than to bring down a dangerously high blood glucose level—provided treatment is started in time.

What is lactic acidosis (LA)?

Lactic acidosis is a condition like DKA that results from a metabolic imbalance. Lactic acid is normally present in blood and muscle tissue as a byproduct of the metabolism of glucose. When some event such as a heart attack limits oxygen to the blood and tissues, lactic acid levels can build up. LA occurring with diabetes is rare. The symptoms can be like those of DKA. The high blood acid level causes nausea and vomiting, and the patient has to breathe hard (hyperventilate) to get rid of the carbon dioxide being released.

Who is at risk for developing LA?

Rarely, lactic acidosis will appear in people with type 2 diabetes who take metformin, an oral antidiabetic medication. Metformin (Glucophage) has a different structure and different modes of action from sulfonylurea drugs such as glyburide and glipizide. It is an effective and safe agent for the control of hyperglycemia in people with type 2 diabetes. However, if the kidney is not functioning, problems can arise. For example, JD is taking metformin for his type 2 diabetes. He also has vascular disease and had dye-contrast X rays taken yesterday. Today the dye is causing kidney problems. Because he was not told to stop the metformin before the test, he develops LA.

Although LA is an uncommon complication of taking metformin, it does happen. **You should not be taking metformin if you have kidney disease, liver disease, alcoholism, cardiovascular disease, or if you are pregnant.** If you have none of these diseases, are not pregnant, and are taking metformin, report promptly symptoms of nausea, vomiting, abdominal pain, lethargy, or hyperventilation to your physician.

What are the symptoms of LA?

The symptoms of lactic acid poisoning are shock, severe anemia, low blood pressure, and hyperventilation. LA can have serious effects on the heart and blood circulation, affecting heart rhythm, heart rate, and blood pressure.

What is the treatment for LA?

As with DKA, it is important to restore circulation and provide sufficient oxygen and nutrients to all the body tissues. Saline (salt and water) may be given intravenously along with sodium bicarbonate (a sterile form of baking soda) to neutralize the acid in the blood. Using a dialysis machine to cleanse the blood of metformin and lactic acid is sometimes an effective and successful treatment, restoring metabolic balance in the tissues.

In conclusion

These descriptions of the acute complications of diabetes are meant to be informational and not alarming. With prompt recognition of these complications, they can be treated effectively, and in most instances, the outcome is good. Failure to recognize the true situation in time and thus delay in getting prompt medical treatment are the major reasons for a poor outcome. As with every aspect of diabetes, you and your family are full and equal partners in the diabetes care team. Your knowledge and participation are vital if you are to live in comfortable equilibrium with your disease.

This chapter was written by Saul M. Genuth, MD.

2

Hypoglycemia

Hypoglycemia is a side effect of the treatment of diabetes. It is an abnormally low level of glucose in the blood.

How does the body regulate the amount of glucose in the blood?

In a person who does not have diabetes, blood glucose levels are regulated precisely and kept within a narrow range. For a person to develop significant hypoglycemia, something must go wrong with these regulatory mechanisms.

Although we eat a variety of natural sugars in our diets, all of them must be broken down into glucose before they can be absorbed from the intestines into the blood. Only glucose is utilized by the cells of the body, and it needs insulin to get into the cells.

Your level of blood glucose at any moment reflects a balance among the amount of glucose absorbed from the intestine, that released from the liver into the blood, and that exiting from the blood into the various cells of the body (Figure 2-1). The glucose that comes from the liver actually has two sources within the liver: *1*) that released from storage in the cells of the liver (the storage form of glucose is called *glycogen*), a process called *glycogenolysis;*

and *2)* that converted from protein and other substances, a process called *gluconeogenesis* (new glucose formation). These processes are blocked when a lot of insulin is in your blood, and conversely, they release glucose rapidly when blood insulin levels are low.

The rise in glucose that occurs after a meal stimulates the pancreas islet cells to secrete insulin into the blood. The insulin then allows the glucose to move into the cells, thereby lowering blood glucose levels. As the glucose levels fall, insulin secretion also falls, and this stabilizes the blood glucose levels before they get too low.

Although insulin is the only hormone that directly promotes glucose uptake by cells and lowers blood glucose levels (Figure 2-1), there are several other body hormones—*glucagon, epinephrine, cortisol,* and *growth hormone*—that work in the opposite fashion. They raise glucose levels (Table 2-1). All of these hormones are released into the blood when you get hypoglycemic, and together they are referred to as *counterregulatory* or *stress hormones.*

Glucagon is made in the islets of the pancreas, as is insulin, but in a different type of cell. The islet alpha cells make glucagon, and the islet beta cells make insulin. Glucagon powerfully stimulates both glycogenolysis and gluconeogenesis in the liver, and it raises glucose levels within a few minutes.

Epinephrine, also known as adrenaline, is made by the adrenal glands, which are located in the abdomen above the kidneys. Epinephrine also stimulates glycogenolysis and gluconeogenesis and also works within minutes. More delayed effects of epinephrine include suppressing insulin release and causing the cells not to respond well to insulin. Epinephrine also affects the heart and nervous system. When it is released because of hypo-

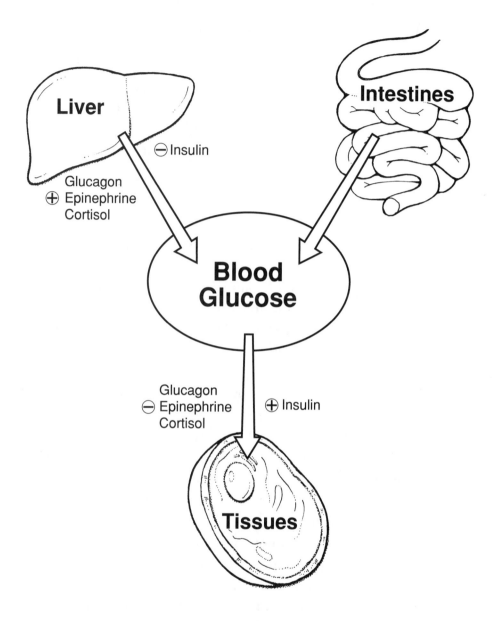

Figure 2-1. Glucose can enter the blood from the intestines after food is digested and from the liver either by breakdown of stored glycogen (glycogenolysis) or by formation from other substances (gluconeogenesis). Glucose release from the liver is increased when glucagon, epinephrine, and cortisol levels in the blood are elevated and is decreased when insulin levels in the blood are high. Glucose exits out of the blood into the various tissues of the body, a process made possible by insulin and partially blocked by cortisol, epinephrine, and growth hormone.

Table 2-1. Hormones Controlling Glucose Levels

Lower Glucose Levels	Raise Glucose Levels
Insulin	Glucagon
	Epinephrine (adrenaline)
	Cortisol
	Growth hormone

glycemia, it causes a rapid heartbeat, sweating, and a feeling of anxiety.

Cortisol is released by another part of the adrenal glands and acts more slowly to raise blood glucose levels through stimulating gluconeogenesis and causes the cells to respond less efficiently to insulin. *Growth hormone* is released by the pituitary gland, which sits under the brain. It also acts more slowly to raise blood glucose levels by causing the cells to respond less efficiently to insulin.

In addition to cortisol and growth hormone release, there are a number of other conditions that decrease the cells' sensitivity to insulin, a condition known as *insulin resistance.* With insulin resistance, there are usually large amounts of insulin in the blood; however, the insulin is ineffective. It can't lower blood glucose, because the cells are resistant to its action. Conditions that lead to insulin resistance include obesity, age, infections, and certain medications. People with type 2 diabetes generally tend to be much more insulin resistant and are less likely to develop hypoglycemia than people with type 1 diabetes.

What are the symptoms of hypoglycemia?

Symptoms of hypoglycemia are usually divided into those that affect the body and those that affect the brain (Table

Table 2-2. Symptoms of Hypoglycemia

Bodily Symptoms	Central Nervous System Symptoms
Rapid heartbeat	Light-headedness
Sweating	Confusion
Tremors	Headache
Anxiety	Loss of consciousness (coma)
Hunger	Seizures
Nausea	Delayed reflexes
	Slurred speech

2-2). Among the bodily symptoms, rapid and forceful heartbeat, hunger, sweating, nausea, and headache are the most common. Most of these symptoms are related to the release of epinephrine.

When the brain is affected, symptoms may range from light-headedness and anxiety to confusion, loss of consciousness, and even seizures. These symptoms are directly related to the brain's not receiving enough glucose for use as an energy source. The bodily symptoms usually develop over several minutes, and their severity depends on both how low the glucose levels go and how rapidly they are falling.

What is hypoglycemia unawareness?

People who have many hypoglycemic episodes may just feel a bit strange and have to sense that they are "low" without more specific symptoms. Sometimes they lose all of the warning symptoms, and the first symptom is that they become confused. This is referred to as *hypoglycemia unawareness* and is a potentially dangerous situation because hypoglycemic confusion can occur without warning. If you are driving a car or operating heavy machinery, even the slightest bit of confusion or delayed reaction may cause an accident.

Some people develop hypoglycemia unawareness **because** they have lots of hypoglycemic episodes. The body has gradually adapted to the hypoglycemia so that it takes a lower and lower blood glucose level to cause a release of epinephrine and the associated warning symptoms. However, the brain does not adapt, and the glucose level that causes warning symptoms becomes lower than the level that causes confusion. Frequent hypoglycemic episodes cause hypoglycemia unawareness, and the unawareness makes the person susceptible to even more hypoglycemia—a vicious cycle.

In people who have long-standing type 1 diabetes and diabetic neuropathy (nerve damage) that involves the internal organs (called autonomic neuropathy), epinephrine is not released when it should be, thus preventing the warning symptoms from developing. In most of these people, glucagon is also not released from the pancreas, so the immediate counterregulatory hormone response is lost, and hypoglycemia may last longer (see chapter 12).

If you have hypoglycemia unawareness, you may lose the early symptoms of hypoglycemia, although others may notice that you are pale, have slurred speech, aren't making sense, or are irritable even though you feel fine. Because you don't know you need to treat the reaction, you are at risk of letting your blood glucose become so low that you pass out.

If you have hypoglycemia unawareness, testing your blood glucose levels frequently and wearing diabetes identification are of particular importance for your safety. Always test your blood glucose before you drive and every

1–2 hours on extended trips. You need to do what your body used to do for you to protect yourself and others.

Are there different levels of hypoglycemia?

You can define different levels of hypoglycemia based on the severity of the symptoms and whether you need help from another person. Mild hypoglycemia is when you recognize the symptoms and can treat the low blood glucose yourself. With moderate hypoglycemia, your symptoms are more severe, your thinking is impaired, and you have difficulty managing it yourself and need help from someone else. With severe hypoglycemia, you may suddenly lose consciousness or have seizures; you must have assistance. Hypoglycemia unawareness is true hypoglycemia, but you are aware of no symptoms. Pseudo-hypoglycemia occurs when you have signs and symptoms of hypoglycemia but actually have a normal blood glucose level. This happens often in people who have had high blood glucose for long periods and suddenly decrease into normal ranges, which results in a surge of regulatory hormones.

Do people without diabetes develop hypoglycemia?

Hypoglycemia is extremely rare in healthy individuals. Even if someone fasts for 3 days with no glucose coming in from food, glucose levels fall somewhat but not to hypoglycemic levels. The liver still produces a small amount of glucose (gluconeogenesis), and the pancreas doesn't produce insulin because of the lower level of glucose, so glucose uptake into cells is decreased markedly. With more prolonged starvation, glucose levels may dip below 50 mg/dl, but this rarely happens outside of countries plagued by malnutrition.

In some people, glucose may be more rapidly absorbed from the intestine, triggering a rise in insulin. Then, while the elevated insulin levels are sending glucose into the cells, no more glucose is coming in from the intestine, and there is an imbalance. Hypoglycemia can occur. However, this hypoglycemia is usually limited—lasting only a few minutes up to an hour or two—because the counterregulatory hormones discussed above get released and stimulate the liver to release more glucose into the blood. Besides, the low glucose levels have shut off further insulin release so that as soon as the insulin itself is metabolized (something that occurs in 30–60 minutes), it is no longer stimulating glucose uptake by the cells.

Treatment for this type of hypoglycemia involves avoiding a lot of concentrated sweets at main meals to decrease the rise in blood glucose and consequent rise in secreted insulin. Occasionally, people have small snacks between meals to match the time that insulin is causing glucose levels to decrease. Treatment to delay stomach emptying, such as eating foods high in insoluble fiber, may be helpful, and taking medications such as oral diazoxide is sometimes useful.

What is the treatment for hypoglycemia in patients with type 2 diabetes treated with diet and exercise alone?

In some people with type 2 diabetes, the body is still making an adequate amount of insulin, but its glucose-stimulated release may be delayed by several minutes. In this way, insulin levels may still be high after the ingestion of glucose from a meal is complete (similar to what happens in the healthy individual with rapid intestinal absorption discussed above). Again the treatment is to avoid concentrated sweets at main meals and to have between-meal snacks. Treatment to delay stomach emptying may prove useful in some patients, and others may benefit from medications that delay glucose absorption, such as acarbose and miglitol.

What is the treatment for hypoglycemia in people with type 2 diabetes who are taking oral medications for their diabetes?

Sulfonylureas

Sulfonylurea is the name given to the class of medications that treat diabetes by stimulating insulin release by the pancreas. Table 2-3 lists these medications, which can cause both brief and more prolonged hypoglycemia.

The brief or transient hypoglycemia is rare but may occur 2–3 hours after a meal and is the result of the sulfonylurea causing too much insulin to be released from the pancreas. It is usually caused by skipping a meal or taking too much medication. This hypoglycemia is usually mild and self-limited. Usually you detect it either by symptoms or by self-monitoring blood glucose (SMBG) and

Table 2-3. Oral Medications Used to Treat Diabetes

Sulfonylureas	Insulin Facilitators	Alter Glucose Absorption
First generation	Metformin (Glucophage)	Acarbose (Precose)
Tolbutamide (Orinase)	Troglitazone (Rezulin)	Miglitol
Chlorpropamide (Diabinase)		
Tolazamide (Tolinase)		
Second generation		
Glyburide (Diabeta, Micronase, Glynase)		
Glipizide (Glucotrol, Glucotrol XL)		
Glimepiride (Amaryl)		

getting a low reading between meals. This type of hypo-glycemia is usually easily treated by reducing the dose of medication. You may also have a small snack between meals. Medication such as acarbose or miglitol may be given to you to delay glucose absorption from the intestines so there'll be a closer match between insulin release and glucose absorption times.

The more prolonged hypoglycemia due to oral sul-fonylurea agents is much less common and is seen mainly in people taking the longer-acting medications chlor-propamide and glyburide who have kidney failure or renal impairment. They should use caution when taking these drugs. The prolonged hypoglycemic episodes also occur more commonly in older individuals, who may skip meals. The hypoglycemia may last for many hours and even longer than a day. Treatment consists of eating immediately, but hospitalization may be necessary because of the prolonged nature of the hypoglycemia.

Other oral agents—metformin, acarbose, miglitol, troglitazone

People who take metformin (Glucophage), acarbose (Pre-cose), and troglitazone (Rezulin) should not experience hypoglycemia when these drugs are used alone. However, when any of these medications is used in combination with a sulfonylurea or with insulin, hypoglycemia may occur. As noted above, hypoglycemia occurring in some-one being treated with acarbose or miglitol must be treated with pure glucose tablets and not candy, juice, or table sugar.

What causes hypoglycemia in people taking insulin?

This is the most common variety of hypoglycemia and results from taking too much insulin, eating too little food, skipping a meal, or exercising without preparation. Because there is always too much insulin under these cir-

Table 2-4. Types of Insulin

Type	Onset (h)	Peak (h)	Duration (h)	Max
Lispro	5–15 min	0.5–1.5	2–4	4–6
Regular	0.5–1	2–3	3–6	6–10
NPH	2–4	4–10	10–16	14–18
Lente	3–4	4–12	12–18	16–20
Ultralente	6–10	–	18–20	20–24

Note: The doses of insulin given before each meal increase with higher glucose readings before that meal. These doses are further adjusted by the anticipated meal size, carbohydrate content of the meal, and any planned exercise to be done. *This insulin algorithm is just an example of what can be done.*

cumstances, the liver does not release glucose and therefore does not play a role early in this process.

Although the usual times of insulin onset of action, peak action, and offset of action can be seen in Table 2-4, it is important to realize that these times are approximate and can vary immensely from one person to another. There can even be variation in the same individual depending on where the insulin is injected—absorption is fastest from the abdomen, intermediate from the arms, and slowest from the thighs and buttocks—and whether there is any scar tissue at the site of injection. If you are exercising within 30–60 minutes of the injection, the blood flow to the legs and arms may be increased, resulting in more rapid absorption of the insulin from the site of injection into the blood. On the other hand, if someone mixes a short-acting insulin such as regular with an intermediate-acting insulin such as lente or NPH or a longer-acting insulin such as ultralente in the same syringe, some of the regular will turn into long-acting insulin if the mixture is allowed to stay in the syringe longer than 5 minutes before injection.

What is the treatment for hypoglycemia if you take insulin?

The best treatment for hypoglycemia related to insulin use is to avoid it by planning food, insulin dose, and exercise. For example, if you know you are going to exercise after school or after work, you should adjust for the insulin-sensitizing effect of exercise by decreasing your insulin dose or by eating a snack. The precise amount to lower insulin or to eat extra food for a given amount of exercise is something that you have to work out for yourself with guidance from your health care providers. Testing your blood glucose before you exercise is very important. Knowing how long your insulin has an affect on you is important so that you can make adjustments to insulin at different times of the day. Frequent SMBG will help you discover these trends and catch a falling blood glucose before it causes symptoms.

How do you adjust insulin and food for exercise?

Let's look at a case study of how insulin and food should be adjusted for exercise. A 16-year-old patient who takes about 12 units of NPH in the morning before breakfast and 8 units of NPH before supper uses a sliding scale for his insulin regimen based on his blood glucose reading before each meal (Table 2-5). On days when he knows he has basketball practice after school, he lowers his morning dose of NPH by 4 units and his evening dose of NPH by 2 units. He also decreases his lunch regular insulin by 2 units and his supper regular insulin by 1 unit. He has learned that this is what is necessary to prevent hypoglycemia from occurring during practice and later that evening. Most people don't realize that exercise some-

Table 2-5. Example of Insulin Algorithm

Glucose Level	Regular Insulin Doses at Each Meal		
	Breakfast	Lunch	Supper
Less than 100	5	4	7
101–150	6	5	8
151–200	7	6	9
201–250	8	7	10
251–300	9	8	11
301–350	10	9	12
351–400	11	10	13
More than 400	12	11	14

Note: *This insulin algorithm is just an example of what can be done, and an individually developed algorithm must be developed for each person. The doses of insulin given before each meal increase with higher glucose readings before that meal. These doses are further adjusted by the anticipated meal size, carbohydrate content of the meal, and any planned exercise to be done.*

The doses of regular insulin are given in addition to intermediate- or long-acting insulins given once or twice a day.

times has a prolonged effect in lowering glucose levels—up to 24 hours. Knowing that the effect can last that long, he'll eat a bigger bedtime snack than usual. He also carries glucose tablets with him in case his game is more vigorous or longer than he expected so that he can treat unexpected hypoglycemia.

What else can you do to treat hypoglycemia?

Eating food with glucose in it is the most common way to treat a low blood glucose reaction. As little as 15–20 grams of carbohydrate is usually enough (Table 2-6). A candy bar, while more tasty, is really no better and has far more calories! You have to remember that it takes at least 10–15 minutes before what you have eaten appears in your blood to raise your glucose levels. When someone

Table 2-6. Examples of Food Containing 20 Grams of Carbohydrate

Glucose tablets	4 tabs
Orange juice	6 oz
Apple juice	6 oz
Milk	14 oz
Lifesavers	7 Lifesavers
Coca-Cola	6 oz

has symptoms of hypoglycemia or finds that s/he is "low" when checking blood glucose, the person needs to eat 15–20 grams of glucose right away and then wait for at least 15–20 minutes. (Because their symptoms of hypoglycemia have not gone away, it is often tempting for people to keep eating until their symptoms disappear.) Check your blood glucose level at the end of the 15–20 minutes to be sure that it has risen enough.

What can you do to prevent hypoglycemia when you are driving?

Check your blood glucose level before driving and every 2 hours on long trips. Know your symptoms of low blood glucose, and always have something to eat in the car. By the time you feel hypoglycemic, your nervous system reaction times are already decreased, your judgment is impaired, and your ability to respond quickly to an emergency situation is very impaired.

You should not just eat quickly, you should pull off the road. Get in the passenger seat, test, eat, and wait at least

20–30 minutes until you are feeling perfectly normal before driving again.

You should keep a supply of glucose tablets in the car, just in case you forget to carry some in your pocket or purse. The last thing to do when you feel "low" is to decide that you are almost home or only a few blocks from a restaurant or convenience store, and drive the rest of the way. That is a sure way to have an accident that could hurt you and others driving near you.

When you have hypoglycemia without symptoms, you may not feel a hypoglycemic reaction creeping up on you and may already be confused or have delayed reaction times. You could start or continue driving without being aware that you are impaired. That is why it is critical for all people with hypoglycemia unawareness to perform SMBG frequently, especially before getting behind the wheel of a car. An accident that occurs because of hypoglycemia cannot be "blamed" on the hypoglycemia. It is your responsibility not to be hypoglycemic when driving.

What should you tell others to do for you if your hypoglycemia is severe?

Sometimes, a reaction may progress too fast or may occur during sleep at night, so that you become unconscious or have a seizure. The rule is: **Never force juice or other foods into the mouth of an unconscious person.** The food or drink is likely to end up in his or her lungs and can cause pneumonia. If you are unconscious or unable to eat, you need an injection of glucagon, the hormone we talked about above. It is important, if you are prone to hypoglycemia, to teach friends or family members how to give glucagon. You might teach them how to inject insulin. Thist way, the psychological barrier to injecting you can be overcome in a nonemergency. situation. In an emergency, they will not hesitate to give you the glucagon. If you do not respond to glucagon, the paramedics should be called. However, use of glucagon has made calls to paramedics and trips to the emergency room unnecessary in many circumstances. Everyone who takes insulin or a sulfonylurea should have a glucagon kit. If you don't, ask your doctor to prescribe it.

What can you do about nighttime hypoglycemia?

Nighttime hypoglycemic reactions can be particularly disturbing. Often, the warning signs are masked by sleep, so you may be confused and thrash about. On the other hand, nighttime reactions may go unnoticed, the only sign being elevated glucose levels in the morning or waking up drenched in sweat. However, you may also remember vivid dreams or nightmares and wake up with a headache in the morning. Sometimes checking blood glucose at 3:00 A.M. will detect middle-of-the-night lows. These nighttime reactions may be eliminated by reducing the evening dose of NPH or lente or by changing the time it is given. If regular insulin is taken at bedtime, the dose must be reduced. A snack at bedtime may also help.

Can hypoglycemia cause permanent damage?

Hypoglycemia should be avoided, but even repeated hypoglycemic episodes do not have any long-term ill effects on brain functioning, as shown by the detailed studies of people participating in the Diabetes Control and Complications Trial (DCCT). Although possible, other harmful effects of severe hypoglycemia such as heart attack or stroke are rare.

Let's take a worst-case scenario. Suppose you were to become unconscious at home alone from taking too much insulin with too little food. What's the worst thing that could happen? Well, you could die or have permanent brain damage as in the Sonny von Bulow case, but this rarely happens. It is much more likely that you would be unconscious several minutes or up to a few hours. But then, the body's counterregulatory hormones would be released and cause your glucose levels to rise. The insulin that was injected would be metabolized by the body (remember that regular insulin has to be taken several times a day because it doesn't last very long) so that it could no longer produce hypoglycemia. Then, your glucose levels would rise and you would wake up.

Are there other situations in which hypoglycemia can occur?

Some special circumstances for people who take insulin must be considered if hypoglycemia is to be avoided. The most important of these is excessive drinking of alcohol. Alcohol can impair the ability of the liver to form glucose and get it into the blood. If you take your insulin and drink alcohol but don't eat, hypoglycemia is going to happen. Certainly you may have alcohol—but in moderation and always with food.

One special circumstance is travel abroad. If you use insulin, take enough insulin and syringes with you—and have a way to properly dispose of them—as well as a letter from your physician stating that you have diabetes and the syringes are necessary for your treatment. You may also want a prescription for any medications you need in case you run out or lose them on your trip. Be aware that the insulin you buy in other countries may not be the same concentration as the insulin you are used to. Most insulin in the U.S. is the same strength: U-100. This means that it has 100 units of insulin in every cubic centimeter (cc) of fluid. Insulin syringes also come in different sizes that match the strength of insulin. You will need a U-40 syringe to use the U-40 insulin found in Latin America and Europe. Your doctor can help you adjust your dosage so you are taking the right amount.

Another special circumstance is a person who has developed damage to the nerves controlling stomach emptying (called *gastroparesis*, see chapter 13). In such people, emptying of food from the stomach is delayed so that insulin is acting before the stomach has emptied into the small intestine and glucose has been absorbed. This may result in hypoglycemia soon after eating in someone taking regular or lispro insulin. Lispro insulin usually acts quickly, before any glucose is available in people with this condition. People with gastroparesis may need to take their rapid-acting insulin later—sometimes after the meal. Medications to speed stomach emptying may also help.

Another special circumstance is the person who is taking a beta blocker. Common beta blockers include pro-pranolol, metoprolol, and atenolol. These medications are valuable in the treatment of coronary heart disease (angina and after heart attacks), hypertension, and certain heart-rhythm disturbances. Beta blockers block the action of epinephrine that has been released because of hypoglycemia, which prevents many of the warning symptoms from happening. Such a blockade may impair the ability of the liver to release glucose. That is why people who are prone to hypoglycemia but have not had a heart attack should avoid beta blockers. If you must use beta blockers because of heart disease, your blood glucose goals should be raised to avoid hypoglycemia.

Some drug interactions can cause or worsen hypoglycemia. Possible drug interactions should be discussed with your provider.

Finally, remember that exercise will lower blood glucose on its own. Therefore, food, insulin, and oral agents must be balanced in amount and time of administration with the type, amount, and extent of exercise.

What can you learn from a hypoglycemic reaction?

When a severe reaction does occur, analyze it to determine why it happened. Did it occur because a meal was delayed? Did it occur because the dose of insulin was too large? Did it occur because exercise had an unexpected affect? You should always carry something with you to treat a reaction—you shouldn't have to stop to buy something. Glucose tablets don't taste very good, so you don't munch on them as you might if you had some candy in your pocket, and they are pure glucose without the extra calories of fructose. The glucose is quickly absorbed. Hard candies are not recommended for treating hypoglycemia.

In conclusion

We try to approximate what the islet cells do by giving oral medications and insulin, but mismatches between medications, food, and exercise occasionally result in hypoglycemia. You need to find the causes of hypoglycemia in your case, especially the severe reactions. Although long-term harmful effects are rare, severe reactions are very unpleasant and dangerous if they occur while you're driving or responsible for young children. Frequent SMBG is helpful, and prompt treatment of even mild reactions usually prevents them from becoming severe.

This chapter was written by Mark E. Molitch, MD.

3

Feet

Stop it at the start, it's late for medicine to be
prepared when disease has grown strong through
long delays.

Ovid, 43 B.C.–17 A.D.
Remedia Amoris, 91

Introduction

Foot problems are one of the leading causes of hospitalization for the 16 million people with diabetes in the U.S.
It has been estimated that 15% of all people with diabetes
will develop a serious foot problem at some time that can
potentially threaten their limb or even their life. The
most common of these problems are foot deformities,
ulceration, infection, and gangrene (death of the tissue),
which can lead, in the most severe of cases, to amputation of a toe, foot, or leg. Amputation due to gangrene is
one of the most feared of all diabetic complications, with
many patients retaining vivid memories of a relative with
diabetes who had lost a limb after developing a foot infection.

The good news is that you can prevent most ulcers and
thus amputations through daily foot inspection and care,
regular visits to your physician and podiatrist, foot-care
education, wearing proper shoes, and early recognition

and treatment of any suspected trouble areas. Of course, this can only be accomplished if **you** do it, and get the help of your health care providers.

You should have a yearly foot examination, a time for you and your physician to identify any foot deformities that might put you at risk for foot ulcers. If the bones in your feet are moving out of their correct position or causing your foot to change shape, you can be referred to a foot-care specialist before serious problems develop. It is much harder to save a foot when it has been ravaged by infection, vascular disease, and nerve damage. The "stop it at the start" philosophy is as practical today as it was in Ovid's time.

The foot is a marvelously intricate biomechanical structure composed of 26 bones, 23 joints, and 42 muscles. When these structures work together normally, your feet feel great. However, when all of the parts don't work together, problems develop. Common adult foot ailments include corns, calluses, ingrown toenails, bunions, hammertoes, claw toes, arthritis, and limited joint motion. Less common is collapse of the arch, or Charcot's joint.

What are the statistics for diabetes-related amputations?

Recent data indicate that lower-extremity amputations are one of the most common complications of diabetes, totaling between 50,000 and 56,000 cases per year. In fact, approximately 50% of all amputations performed in the U.S. that are not the direct result of trauma occur in patients with diabetes. Lower-extremity amputation rates increase in elderly patients with diabetes and are almost twice as high in men as in women.

There are also differences in these rates for people of various ethnic backgrounds. Among African Americans with diabetes, the rate of amputation is 1.5–2.5 times higher than in Caucasians with diabetes. In certain Hispanic and American Indian populations, these rates can be even higher.

Tragically, after undergoing a major lower-extremity amputation, only 50% of patients survive for 3 years, while the 5-year survival rate is only about 40%. In addition, half of those patients undergoing an amputation of one limb will develop a serious lesion in the other leg within 2 years. Considered together with the estimated medical-care costs of amputations in the U.S. in excess of $1 billion per year, the magnitude of diabetic foot disease and necessity for prevention is clear.

In fact, at least 50% of amputations in people with diabetes can be prevented through appropriate medical care and patient education focusing on foot care. Because most limbs lost in diabetes are the result of nonhealing foot ulcers, you should learn about the nature of these ulcers and how to treat and prevent them.

Is there one cause for the foot problems that lead to amputations?

Foot problems in people with diabetes are usually the result of four primary factors: neuropathy (diminished sensation), poor circulation, and a decreased ability to fight infection. Add to those foot deformities and trauma (injury)—the link between neuropathy or poor circulation and infection. (See Table 3-1.)

Neuropathy

Sensorimotor neuropathy causes a loss of feeling in the feet and legs. You may have numbness or tingling in your toes and feet, and you may not be able to feel where your feet are. Neuropathy allows painless injuries such as blisters or the penetration of foreign bodies (for example, a tack or splinter) to go unnoticed and untreated for a long time. Continued walking on the injured or infected foot results in further trauma and injury.

Sensorimotor neuropathy can also affect the nerves supplying the muscles in your feet and legs. This motor neuropathy can result in muscle weakness or loss of tone in the thighs, legs, and feet and the development of hammertoes, bunions, or other foot deformities. Symptoms can also include pain, numbness, and tingling in the legs and feet (see chapter 11).

Poor circulation

People with diabetes often have circulation disorders in their legs and feet due to atherosclerosis and blockage of arteries. A common symptom of *peripheral vascular disease* is tightness in the calf or buttocks when walking. This is called *intermittent claudication.* Peripheral vascular disease can progress to severe cramping or pain at night or at rest. There may be color and temperature changes (the feet may turn bright red when hanging down and constantly feel cold). Also, the skin may become shiny, thin, and easily damaged, and hair growth may be reduced.

Reduced blood flow to the feet means that they don't get enough oxygen or nutrients they need for maintenance and repair. This becomes critical when the foot is injured, infected, or ulcerated because healing will be slow or not happen at all. Peripheral vascular disease, a major cause of lower-extremity amputation, can often be corrected by vascular bypass operations (see chapter 10).

Infection

People with diabetes are more likely to have infections than people without diabetes and less likely to have a strong immune response to the infection. Thus, infections can rapidly worsen and often go undetected, especially in the presence of neuropathy or vascular disease

Table 3-1. Risk Factors for Diabetic Foot Ulceration

Intrinsic Factors	Extrinsic Factors
Neuropathy	**Minor trauma**
Sensory: loss of sensation	High plantar pressures: excessive callus
Motor: muscle weakness	Shoe pressure: blisters
Vascular disease	Injury: cuts, lacerations, etc.
Ischemia: inadequate circulation	**Thermal injury**
Absent or diminished pulses	Burns from hot soaks, scalds, etc.
Difficulty healing	Frostbite
Susceptibility to infection	**Chemical burns: "corn cures"**
Structural deformity	**Bathroom surgery on ingrown toenails, calluses, etc.**
Previous ulceration	
	Poor knowledge of diabetes
	Cigarette smoking

(poor circulation). Often, the only sign of a developing infection is unexplained high blood sugar levels, even in the absence of fever. In fact, the combination of fever and high blood sugar levels often warns of a severe infection.

When a patient who has had a chronic foot ulcer for several months suddenly develops a fever and flu-like symptoms, it is often mistaken for the flu rather than the spreading of the foot infection. Such infections must be aggressively treated with hospitalization, drainage procedures, and antibiotics to avoid gangrene. In fact, delays in treatment can lead to greater tissue damage and make local toe, partial foot, or even entire foot amputations necessary. Less serious infections can often be treated on an outpatient basis with home care, rest, not bearing weight on the foot, and oral antibiotics. However, the foot must be closely monitored to ensure that the infection improves with such treatment.

Foot deformities

Foot deformities such as hammertoes, bunions, and metatarsal disorders are common in the general population, but have a special significance for people with diabetes (Figure 3-1). When neuropathy or poor circulation is present, these deformities cause pressure lesions (corns, calluses, blisters, ulcers) from ill-fitting shoes or simply walking. Serious infections can result if these lesions go untreated.

A deformed foot requires a specially molded shoe. The role of improper, ill-fitting shoes is emphasized by Dr. Paul Brand, who said, "When a person with diabetes complains that his shoes are killing him, he may very well be correct."

How do foot deformities put your feet at risk for developing ulcers?

It isn't just that your shoes don't fit right. It's more a matter of your bones not being where they're supposed to be. Structural deformities of the foot and ankle contribute to increased pressure and irritation of the skin over the protruding bony areas, which cause skin damage and lead to infection. Your earliest symptoms may be a slight reddening or thickening of the skin (corn or callus) beneath the ball of your foot or on your toes. You repeatedly stress these areas as you walk, and this may result in the formation of open sores (ulcers) and fractures that can lead to serious complications. Ulcers can occur under any of the metatarsal heads (the long bones of the foot extending to the toes), at the tips of the toes, over the tops of the toes, or over any bone prominence. Prompt attention to these conditions is essential.

There is a relationship between body weight and elevated pressure on the foot—it is greater in those who are overweight—but far more important is the presence of bony deformity. Pressure on normal bones does not do the same damage as pressure on deformed ones.

What are some of the more common foot deformities?

The following deformities can lead to the development of foot complications.

Hammertoes

A hammertoe is a flexible or rigid deformity characterized by buckling of the toe. The toe takes on the configu-

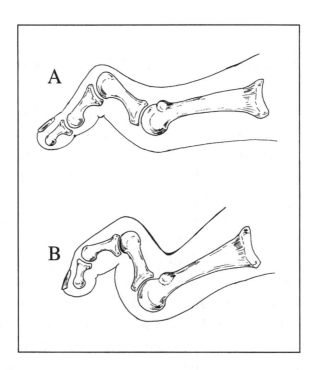

Figure 3-1. A. Hammertoe. B. Claw toe.

ration of a swan's neck. This condition is frequently associated with a bunion deformity. In people with diabetes
and neuropathy, hammertoes are commonly caused by
weakness of the small muscles of the foot, which can't stabilize the toes on the ground. Muscle imbalance results in
the affected toe sitting slightly back and up on the
metatarsal head. This deformity results in increased pressure on the ball of the foot, with irritation at the tip and
top of the toe (Figure 3-1). Hammertoes cause problems
with shoe fitting, because they require more room in the
front (toe box) of the shoe. Improperly fitting shoes
cause rubbing at the top of the toe and may result in an
ulcer.

Claw toes

Claw toes are similar to hammertoes but with more buckling and greater deformity. There is marked flexion of
the toe at its first and second joints. The affected toes sit
on top of their respective metatarsal heads and push
down on the ball of the foot. Claw toes are usually seen
on feet with high arches, but they also occur independently. As with hammertoes, shoe fitting is difficult and
requires a deep toe box.

Prominent metatarsal heads

The metatarsals are the five long bones located in the
mid- and forefoot, just behind the toes. The metatarsal
heads, which are similar in appearance to the knuckles of
the hand, are located in the ball of the foot and support
the body's weight. Normally, these bones share weight
evenly across the ball of the foot. However, if one
metatarsal bone is longer or lower than its adjacent
neighbors, it carries a disproportionate amount of weight.
This can result in pain, callus formation, and ulceration
of the foot.

Bunions (hallux valgus)

A bunion is an enlargement of bone at the base of the big toe joint. Bunions are not caused by tight shoes, and, most often, they are an inherited characteristic. In this condition, the big toe angles toward the second toe and may underlap or override the second toe (Figure 3-2). When the foot is forced into a tight shoe, there is pressure over the prominent first metatarsal head, which can result in an ulcer. Arthritis may be associated with bunions, resulting in pain and stiffness of the joint. Restricted motion in the big toe joint results in the formation of a callus or ulcer beneath the big toe.

Limited joint motion and hallux limitus

Limited motion in the joints of the foot and ankle may lead to abnormal pressure and subsequent skin damage on the bottom of the foot. A common arthritic condition affecting the big toe joint is hallux limitus. This disorder is characterized by degenerative arthritis with limited motion of the big toe joint (first metatarsal phalangeal joint). The big toe is unable to bend normally as the heel lifts off the ground, and the body's weight shifts to the ball of the foot. The result of this limited joint motion is increased pressure beneath the big toe (hallux) and subsequent callus formation, followed by ulceration.

Partial foot amputation

Surgery can "create" a foot deformity, and like any other deformity, it puts unusual pressure on the bones in the foot. Although surgical removal of one or more toes or a major part of the foot may be necessary to save the foot, it increases the risk for future ulceration and amputation. Transmetatarsal amputation (TMA) is done through the metatarsal bones. In essence, the forefoot is amputated.

This surgery provides good future functioning of the foot in terms of flexibility and mobility, and patients seem satisfied with the long-term results. Although TMA shortens the foot, it preserves foot function, is cosmetically acceptable, does not require a prosthesis, and fits well with therapeutic footwear. However, padding is necessary in the shoe to fill the gap from the amputated part of the foot. Proper fitting should be done with the help of a health care professional familiar with this process.

If you ever have an amputation, you will need time to adjust. Physical therapy can help with strength and mobility. You may be surprised by the emotions you feel. Talking with a counselor or a support group can help you regain your emotional balance.

Charcot's joints

Charcot's (shar-kos) joints are an uncommon but potentially serious complication of diabetes. This disorder is characterized by the sudden and unexpected development of redness, swelling, increased warmth, mild to moderate aching, and an inability to fit into your regular shoes. If this should happen, stay off the foot, and see your provider at once because several weeks or months later, the arch will collapse. You may have good circulation and strong pulses in the foot, but you probably have loss of feeling. Most people go to their doctor with the chief complaint that their foot is red and swollen. From a seemingly minor injury may come a cascade of events that result ultimately in severe fractures and dislocations of multiple joints in the middle of the foot and ankle. When the middle of the foot has collapsed, there is deformity, with a rocker-bottom configuration of the foot and increased pressure on the bottom of the foot. This often results in ulceration of the skin. The foot can become so deformed that walking is difficult. Special footwear is very important for this condition.

Who is most at risk for Charcot's joint?

People at high risk for this condition generally have had diabetes for more than 10 years, have loss of sensation in their feet, and are in their 50s or 60s. Of course, people with type 1 diabetes may be much younger. People who also have complications affecting their eyes, kidneys, and nerves appear to be at greatest risk for the development of bone and joint destruction. These changes may be difficult to distinguish from bone destruction caused by infection. Injury to the foot can put you at risk, as does smoking, living alone, and not having good foot-care training.

What is the treatment for acute onset of Charcot foot?

The treatment is to stop bearing weight on the foot. This can be accomplished by a specially applied cast or other devices. If you are allowed to walk, fractures and the foot deformities noted above are likely to follow.

What are the symptoms of foot problems?

The following warning signs are associated with diabetic foot complications and require prompt evaluation and treatment by a foot-care specialist:

- Redness, swelling, or increased skin temperature of the foot or ankle
- A change in the size or shape of the foot or ankle
- Pain in the legs at rest or while walking
- Open sores with or without drainage, no matter how small
- Nonhealing wounds

- Ingrown toenails
- Corns or calluses with skin discoloration

What treatments are available for foot deformities?

Therapeutic footwear and custom insoles are essential parts of the management program for adults with diabetes. If you have foot deformities or a loss of feeling in your feet, you should have your shoes fitted by a podiatrist who is specially trained in the treatment of diabetic foot disorders; a pedorthist, who is specially trained in fitting therapeutic shoes;, or an orthotist, who specializes in fitting prostheses. If you have hammertoes and prominent metatarsal heads, you can avoid pressure over the protruding joints by wearing extra-depth shoes.

Your prescription footwear needs to offer *1*) relief of pressure, *2*) accommodation of deformities, *3*) support, and *4*) limitation of joint motion in cases where motion is excessive.

How can you detect and prevent foot complications?

The American Diabetes Association recommends that you receive an annual foot examination for assessment of sensation, circulation, foot deformities, and other risk factors for ulceration or amputation. If you have foot deformities, ingrown toenails (or other toenail problems), ulcers, corns, or calluses, they should be evaluated by a person who specializes in treatment and preventive foot care. You may need surgery for disabling deformities, and your options should be discussed with your physician. For example, hammertoe correction may give you relief of pressure beneath a metatarsal head or over a prominent toe.

Surgery is advised for the treatment of hallux limitus (arthritic condition affecting the joint of the big toe, see above) when it is associated with ulceration beneath the big toe. A surgical procedure that results in increased range of motion of the big toe relieves pressure at the site of the ulcer and helps it heal.

Having good blood sugar control can help delay the onset of neuropathy. Therefore, you would be able to feel an injury to your foot when it happens.

Injury can be avoided by inspecting your feet and the inside of your shoes daily. Do not use "corn cures" or do bathroom surgery on ingrown toenails or calluses. Don't walk barefoot, especially outside, and do wear comfortable socks and cushioned, roomy shoes that do not press against your feet or toes. These are commonsense approaches to prevention that can have great payoffs.

What is an ulcer?

An ulceration, or ulcer, is usually a painless open sore on the bottom of the foot or top or tip of a toe. It results from pressure from your shoes, a corn or callus that has grown too thick, or an injury such as a splinter. Continued walking on the injury creates even further damage. The open sore frequently becomes infected and may even penetrate to the bone.

How can ulcers be treated?

Treatment relies heavily on early recognition of the ulceration, avoidance of walking, and early intervention by your health care provider. Aside from local wound care, dressings, and antibiotics, various other measures may be necessary to adequately relieve pressure on the area. Your physician should evaluate the depth and size of the ulcer and obtain X rays of the foot. X rays help determine whether there is a foreign body in your foot, infection in the bone (osteomyelitis), or any gas or air deep in the tissues. Gas or air in a wound suggests infection. Sometimes, a more sophisticated examination using magnetic resonance imaging (MRI) is necessary. Most ulcers occur over the ball of the foot, on the bottom of the big toe. When an ulcer occurs somewhere else, the physician must be suspicious about what caused it. If it occurs in an unusual place, cannot be explained by injury, and is not responding to treatment, the doctor should consider doing a biopsy. A biopsy consists of surgically removing a small amount of tissue to examine under the microscope for the possibility of a malignancy (cancer).

It is essential that all the dead tissue in an ulcer be removed (debrided). Leaving any dead tissue makes it extremely difficult to heal an infected ulcer. The ulcer may need to be cultured for bacteria.

Controlling your blood sugar is extremely important because high blood sugar interferes with your white blood cells' ability to fight infection. Check your blood sugar at home, and try to keep it as close to normal as possible. Signs of worsening infection are increased redness around the ulcer or red streaks going up your leg. This is evidence of spreading infection and is called *lymphangitis*. If you notice increased drainage and the foot has a bad odor, call your physician at once. If you develop pain or if a foot with an ulcer on the bottom gets red and puffy on the top of the foot, notify your physician, because these are signs of spreading infection. Do not soak your foot. Be very, very careful.

Most important is to stay off the foot. Do not put weight on an ulcerated foot. Walking on an ulcer prevents healing and may actually cause it to become worse. Use crutches, a wheelchair, or bed rest. Later, plaster casts, braces, healing sandals, special shoe inserts, or padding may be used to protect the foot while it heals. If circulation is inadequate for healing, your doctor may refer you to a vascular surgeon for appropriate evaluation and possible vascular reconstructive surgery (see chapter 10).

Why don't some ulcers heal?

Ulcers can take months to heal. During this time, keep your diabetes in good control to allow healing to take place. Your participation in your care is vital, because you treat most ulcers at home with the assistance of family members or visiting nurses.

When ulcers are slow to heal or get worse, several possible causes must be considered. First, some patients don't stay off the foot. If walking or weight bearing is the direct cause of the ulcer, it makes sense that continued walking will prevent it from healing. (You do not cure tennis elbow by continuing to play tennis!) Denial is common, because patients with neuropathy can't feel the

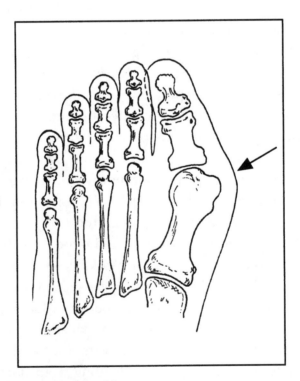

Figure 3-2. A bunion is a significant foot deformity.

The Uncomplicated Guide to Diabetes Complications

sore. If it can't be felt (and isn't seen), it is easy to ignore. Walking continues (without a limp), the pressure continues, and the ulcer does not heal or gets worse. Work-related issues are a significant concern because many patients are unable to take time off from their jobs to allow for proper healing. Wheelchairs or crutches may be necessary.

A second reason for impaired healing can be peripheral vascular disease (ischemia), which prevents the blood from delivering essential nutrients, oxygen, and antibiotics to the ulcerated area. Without adequate blood flow to the foot, the ulcer will not heal. Your physician can check blood pressure at your ankles and arms. They should be the same, and if they are not, you may have blocked arteries in the leg. When significant blockages exist, consultation with a vascular surgeon is recommended. Vascular bypass operations in the legs and feet restore circulation and promote the healing of ulcers (see chapter 10).

Underlying or deep-seated infection is the third major reason many foot ulcers do not heal. Chronic infections often have no symptoms. Constant draining or a discharge from the ulcer may be a sign of an underlying infection. Wound cultures should be taken periodically to assess the bacterial growth in the ulcer and to determine which, if any, of the bacteria need to be treated with antibiotics. Keep in mind, however, that ulcers are rarely sterile, and routine culture obtained by swabbing may not yield the bacteria that is actually causing the infection. Antibiotic treatment based on the false culture results may not help. Tissue obtained from debridement or a punch biopsy may be sent for analysis. If a probe can actually touch bone at the base of the ulcer, it strongly suggests bone infection (osteomyelitis) that will require more aggressive treatment. If you have a long-standing ulcer that suddenly gets worse, associated with fever and elevated blood sugar levels, you will need immediate hospitalization for proper care.

How can you prevent an ulcer from developing?

You don't want an ulcer, and you don't want a healed ulcer to return. Prevention is the key to saving your limbs. Good habits must be developed early and continued for your lifetime. If you are faithful in your foot-care program, your chances for preventing serious foot problems are significantly improved.

There are several key components of the prevention program that can be called the "5 Ps of prevention." They are professional care, protective footwear, pressure reduction, prophylactic surgery, and preventive education (Table 3-2).

Professional care

You need periodic examinations and care by a health care professional familiar with diabetic foot care. In this regard, a podiatrist skilled in diabetic foot care can be an important member of your health care team. A podiatrist can examine your feet and check for neuropathy, circulation problems, and potential trouble spots or trim toenails and calluses before they become problems. Studies have shown that such regular care—at least several times each year—is important in preventing foot problems.

Protective footwear

Much of the minor trauma leading to foot ulceration is a result of improperly fitting shoes. The orthopedist, podiatrist, pedorthist, or orthotist should assist you in selecting and fitting shoes for the shape of your foot and any type of deformity. Walking or athletic shoes are good for most patients; however, several studies have shown that patients with a healed ulcer who wore specially designed shoes (with extra depth for the toes and cushioned soles) were much less likely to get another ulcer than were patients who continued to wear their regular shoes.

Pressure reduction

You can relieve pressure on the soles of your feet by wearing cushioned footwear, padded socks, and insoles. The most common sign of higher-than-normal pressures under an area of the foot is a callus, which is the skin's normal response to excessive pressure. If you reduce the pressure on this part of the foot, you can reduce the size of the callus and possibly prevent an ulcer from developing under it. Most ulcers occur where there is a callus. If the callus comes back after the ulcer heals, there is a strong likelihood of the ulcer coming back, too.

High pressures can be measured by footprint analysis using pressure-sensitive mats or by computerized gait analysis systems. Potential problem areas or "hot spots" can be detected and treated with inserts for your shoes. In-shoe pressure measurements are useful for seeing the effectiveness of the insoles.

Prophylactic surgery

Occasionally, preventive or reconstructive foot surgery stops ulcers from happening by repairing a structural problem in the foot that would eventually cause an ulcer. In addition, reconstructive surgery is often necessary to heal chronic ulcers that don't respond to other treatments. This surgery is done only when arterial disease is not present or has been corrected. These procedures can preserve the weight-bearing function of the foot and avoid the need for amputation. This is not an endorse-

Table 3-2. The 5 Ps of Prevention

1. Professional care

> Regular visits, examinations, and foot care

> Early detection and aggressive treatment of new lesions

2. Protective shoes

> Adequate room to protect from injury, well cushioned

> Walking sneakers, extra-depth or custom-molded shoes

> Special modifications as necessary

3. Pressure reduction

> Cushioned insoles, custom orthotics, padded hosiery

> Pressure measurements, computerized or mat

4. Prophylactic surgery

> Correct structural deformities (hammertoes, bunions, Charcot's joint, etc.)

> Prevent recurrent ulcers over or under deformities

> Intervene early

5. Preventive education

> Patient education: need for daily inspection and early intervention

> Physician education: significance of foot lesions, importance of regular foot examinations, and current concepts in diabetic foot management

ment for the routine correction of any hammertoe or foot deformity. Most problems are best managed by special shoes and pressure-reduction therapies. However, when these treatments are not successful in patients with adequate circulation, it is time to consider corrective foot surgery in selective cases. The decision requires the combined input and cooperation of your family, primary physician, and surgeon. You should avoid unnecessary surgery at all costs. Good postoperative care is critical to the success of surgery and frequently requires special visiting nurses.

Preventive education

Many foot ulcers are caused by external factors, improper self care, or neglect. That is why the foot-care guidance from your diabetes educator, nurse specialist, physician, or podiatrist is so valuable. Nothing is more important than keeping your feet clean and dry and inspecting them every day. Remove both shoes and socks at every doctor's appointment. Take part in diabetic foot-care courses, and learn to recognize potential warning signs. That's how you reduce the risk for foot ulcerations.

Foot care is seldom accomplished by one health care provider. You usually will have a team, depending on the condition of your feet.

Who should see your feet?

Foot problems may require care by your primary care physician, an endocrinologist or diabetologist, a podiatrist, an orthopedic surgeon, a plastic surgeon, a vascular surgeon, a diabetes educator, a wound-care specialist, or a rehabilitation specialist experienced in the management of people with diabetes. These team members should communicate with each other about your condition and treatment. All patients, especially those with loss of sensation, foot deformity, and diminished circulation, should receive a comprehensive foot examination and education about the risks and prevention of foot problems.

What shoes should you wear?

Shoes are meant to protect your feet, not to hurt them. Shoes must always fit comfortably, with adequate length, width, and depth for the toes. If a shoe is hard to put on, don't wear it. It may be too small for your foot and may cause serious damage, especially if you have neuropathy or poor circulation. Shoes should preferably be made of leather, which will easily adapt to the shape of your feet and allow your feet to breathe. Athletic shoes, jogging shoes, and sneakers are excellent choices as long as they are well fitted and provide adequate cushioning. Your doctor may recommend extra-depth shoes or custom molded shoes to accommodate your needs. Also, special insoles or custom orthotics may be prescribed for cushioning and support.

Always look and feel inside your shoes for foreign objects or torn linings before putting them on. You should change your shoes several times a day so that one pair is not worn for more than 4–6 hours. New shoes should be worn only a few hours at a time, and you should inspect your feet for any irritations. Don't break in new shoes: If they don't fit when you try them on in the store, don't buy them. Socks should be well fitted, without seams or folds, and should not be so tight that your circulation is stopped. Well-padded socks can be very protective as long as there is enough room for them in your shoes.

Above all else, do not walk barefooted. Discuss wearing open-toed shoes or sandals with your podiatrist or physician. At the beach or pool, wear protective footwear, especially if you have lost sensation.

What is the correct way to have your shoes fitted?

- Have your feet sized every time you buy shoes. Your feet tend to get longer and wider as you grow older. You might be surprised to find out

what your size is now. And have *both* feet sized—
one may be longer than the other.

- Have your feet measured at the end of the day.
  Feet often swell during the day, and you want to
  buy shoes that will fit *all* day long.
- Keep in mind that sizes vary among different shoe
  brands and styles. Judge the shoe by how it fits,
  not by the size marked in the shoe.
- Once the shoes are on, there should be 3/8 to
  1/2 inch of space beyond your longest toe while
  you're standing; at the same time, the ball of your
  foot should fit well into the widest part of the shoe.
- Walk in the shoes to make sure they fit well. The
  heels should not slip very much. Don't expect
  shoes to stretch to fit. If they aren't comfortable at
  the time of the fitting, don't buy them.

What do you need to know about therapeutic shoes?

People with diabetes who are at risk for amputation can
get special shoes and inserts, and Medicare will pick up
part of the cost. Such therapeutic footwear has been
shown to reduce the risk of foot ulcers that can lead to
amputation. The doctor who is treating you for diabetes
needs to fill out a form certifying that you are in a comprehensive plan of diabetes care, have evidence of diabetic foot disease (nerve damage with calluses, prior ulcer
or amputation, foot deformity, or poor circulation), and
need therapeutic footwear. You are referred to a specialist
who writes the prescription, and then you can take the
prescription to someone who dispenses the shoes.

Congress added this benefit in 1993. Still, many doctors
do not recognize the role therapeutic shoes can play in
preventing amputations in people with diabetes, and they

do not tell patients about this Medicare benefit. The next time you see your doctor, ask for a foot exam. If your doctor concludes that you're at risk for a foot ulcer, and you're covered by Medicare Part B, ask to be certified to receive the therapeutic shoe benefit. Otherwise, see a podiatrist, who can get the completed certificate from your doctor.

Where should you go to buy therapeutic shoes?

Many people go to pedorthists to be fitted with therapeutic shoes. Board-certified pedorthists are trained in foot anatomy and the construction of shoes, shoe modifications, and foot orthotics (inserts). Like a pharmacist, a pedorthist fills the prescription for therapeutic shoes that was written for you.

About half of pedorthists work in orthopedic shoe stores, and half work in foot clinics or orthotic-prosthetic facilities. Either way, you should call for an appointment. If your feet tend to swell during the day, make an afternoon appointment.

It will take about 30 minutes for the pedorthist to measure and fit your feet. Ordinarily, the pedorthist won't charge you for his or her time, just for the shoes and inserts you get.

About 85% of people can be fitted with off-the-shelf shoes. The pedorthist might have the shoes you need in stock or will order them. Off-the-shelf shoes may need some adjustment to fit your needs. The uppers may need to be stretched for prominent toes, wedges and flares can be added to the soles for better stability, and rocker soles or metatarsal bars can be added to reduce pressure on certain areas of the foot. Shoes with laces can be converted to Velcro closure if needed. Lifts are added to the inside or outside of the shoes if your legs are different lengths.

You may need inserts for your shoes. These are also called foot orthoses or orthotics. Inserts can be made of foam, leather, or plastic. Softer designs are recommended for people with diabetes to provide shock absorption and to accommodate any abnormalities of the feet, such as calluses or bones that stick out. If your feet can't fit into standard footwear, the pedorthist can fit you for custom-made shoes. These take 3–6 weeks to make.

What if your new shoes feel too big?

When you first put on your new therapeutic shoes, they might feel too loose. They aren't. There are two reasons for this. First, many of us get fixed on the size we wore when we were 20 years old. Yet most people's feet get bigger as they grow older. Second, many people with diabetes have neuropathy (nerve damage) in their feet. Because of decreased sensation in their feet, shoes that are the right size feel too big, so they wear shoes that are too small.

Wear your new shoes 2 hours on and 2 hours off for 3 days. This allows your feet to get accustomed to the shoes. Then wear them all day. In the evening, check your feet for red spots. If any redness lasts more than 30 minutes to an hour after you've taken off the shoes, tell your pedorthist. He or she will probably want to make further adjustments to the shoes.

Your pedorthist will want to see you again after you've worn the shoes and inserts for 6 months. If the inserts are compressed, you'll be fitted for new ones.

What are the guidelines for good foot care?

- At each doctor's visit, remove your shoes and stockings, and have your feet examined.
- Avoid walking barefoot.

- Look inside your shoes for sharp tacks, rough linings, or foreign objects.
- Wear sensible shoes that are properly fitted.
- Inspect your feet daily for blisters, bleeding, and lesions between toes. Make this part of your ritual.
- Use a mirror to see the bottom of your foot and heel. Ask a family member for help.
- Do not soak your feet.
- Avoid temperature extremes—don't use hot water bottles, heating pads, or electric blankets on your feet. Test bath water with your elbow.
- Wash feet daily with warm, soapy water and dry them well, especially between the toes. Put on clean socks.
- Use moisturizing lotion (whose first ingredient is not alcohol) daily but not between the toes.
- Do not use acids or chemical corn removers.
- Do not perform "bathroom surgery" on corns, calluses, or ingrown toenails.
- Trim your nails following the curve of the toe, and file gently. Have a podiatrist do this if you have difficulty doing it.
- Call your doctor immediately if your foot becomes swollen, red, or painful. Stay off the foot.
- Don't smoke.
- Learn all you can about diabetes and foot care.
- Have regular foot examinations by your physician or podiatrist.

Robert G. Frykberg, DPM, MPH; Lee J. Sanders, DPM; and Roger Marzano, CPO, Cped, contributed to this chapter.

4

Eye Disease

Case study

A 36-year-old man who has had type 1 diabetes for 18 years awakened with blurred vision. Beginning 6 months ago, he noted a web in front of one eye, but it cleared after a few days. It recurred once, 6 weeks ago, and lasted approximately 1 week. This morning, he noted blurred vision. When questioned, he realizes he now has difficulty with depth perception such as when attempting to add cream to his coffee.

The ophthalmologist explains the sudden onset of floating specks may be a harmless alteration in the vitreous gel, the material that fills the globe of the eye. However, in a diabetic patient, there is a possibility the floating specks may be caused by a hemorrhage. A dilated-eye exam will be conducted to evaluate the retina and vitreous gel.

Case study

A 60-year-old woman with a 12-year history of type 2 diabetes reports the gradual onset of blurred vision. She has noted difficulty completing her tasks at work, and her employer has complained that she makes too many mistakes. Stronger reading glasses were of temporary value but no longer help. The ophthalmologist explains there are multiple possible causes for her symptoms, including cataract and diabetic retinopathy. A dilated-eye exam will show the status of her retina and whether a cataract is present.

Examination of her macula with a special lens determines that she has macular swelling. The ophthalmologist explains that a fluorescein angiogram will indicate whether the circulation to the macula is impaired and will allow detection of leaky blood vessels.

Introduction

Diabetes can affect your eyes and vision. Some of these effects are mild or short term, such as the blurred vision that comes with poor blood glucose control. Certain complications, however, can be sight threatening, even when your vision is normal. Diabetes is the leading cause of new-onset legal blindness in the U.S. and other industrialized countries. Most of this blindness can be prevented if you keep your blood sugar levels as close to normal as possible and if you get regular examinations and prompt treatment by a physician with experience in diabetic eye care. Because there is usually no pain associated with diabetic eye disease, most people do not have their eyes examined as often as they should.

Regular, life-long eye care is one of the most important elements of managing your diabetes. **Visit an eye-care specialist once a year even if your vision hasn't changed**. When diabetic eye disease is caught early, treatment can be very successful. Current treatments such as laser surgery can prevent more than 95% of severe vision loss from proliferative diabetic retinopathy (disease of the retina) and more than 50% of moderate vision loss from diabetic macular edema (swelling of the macula, a part of the retina).

Other eye changes that can be caused by diabetes are blurred or fluctuating vision, cataracts, glaucoma, and double vision.

How do you see?

Vision is a highly developed and complex process. For you to be able to see, light must be focused by the cornea and lens of the eye through the vitreous gel that fills the eye and onto the retina in the back of the eye, where it is changed into signals that are carried along nerve fibers within the eye (Figure 4-1). These signals are transmitted through the optic nerve to a rear portion of the brain called the visual cortex. Here, visual signals are processed by the brain as sight. Nerves also control the movement of your eyes, adjust the focus, or alter pupil size.

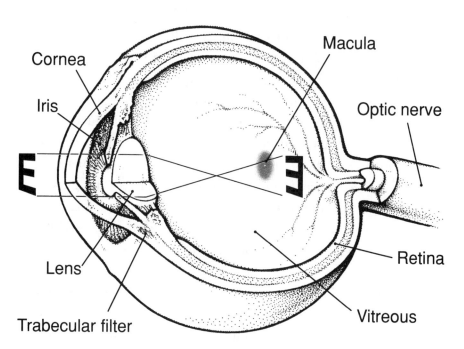

Figure 4-1. Cross-section of an eye indicating the macula, which is responsible for seeing details and color vision.

Any abnormality in the visual system can interfere with your ability to see. For clear vision, there must be no obstruction along the light path within the eye. Scars on the cornea, imperfections in the lens of the eye (such as cataracts), or cloudiness in the vitreous gel of the eye can interfere with light focusing on the retina. The retina is very important to vision. It must be healthy and have a good blood supply, and the nerve transmissions to the brain must go smoothly. The retina can be divided into two zones. The *macula*, or center of the retina, is responsible for detailed central vision that allows you to read, recognize faces, drive, and distinguish colors. The remaining areas of the retina provide peripheral (side) vision, motion detection, and night vision. Obviously, any disease that affects your retina affects your vision. Figure 4-2a (in the color section) shows a normal retina.

How does diabetes affect the retina?

Damage to the retina from diabetes is called *diabetic retinopathy*. The retina consists of many small blood vessels—and uncontrolled blood glucose levels damage small blood vessels. In the eye, this damage changes blood flow and weakens blood vessel walls. The vessel walls can balloon out, allowing fluid or blood to leak into the retina, causing swelling (edema) or leaking (hemorrhages). This is called *nonproliferative* retinopathy. The retina gets less blood and oxygen. This loss of nourishment is called *ischemia*. The affected areas of the retina stop working (Figure 4-2b, in the color section).

If there is no treatment at this point, the eye will compensate. The retina will release growth factors that cause new blood vessels to grow on the retina or on the optic nerve. Although this may seem logical, it often results in devastating complications. The growth of new blood vessels is called *neovascularization* or *proliferative retinopathy*.

The abnormal new vessels are fragile and will bleed and leak. They do not nourish the areas of the eye that have lost circulation and serve no useful purpose (Figure 4-3, in the color section).

New blood vessels growing between the retina and the vitreous gel get pulled and pushed and tend to hemorrhage or leak into the gel. The vitreous gel naturally contracts with aging, but this happens earlier in people with diabetes. If the vitreous detaches before retinopathy develops, you may see a floating line or web, particularly when looking at a bright background, and flashes of light best seen at night. If proliferative retinopathy has begun, the separation of the vitreous gel breaks the blood vessels. Blood flowing into the vitreous gel blocks the path of light, causing you to see floaters, which may vary from a few specks to a dark spot that blocks most of your vision. (Not all floaters indicate proliferative retinopathy.)

Without treatment at this point, scar tissue can develop along these vessels and, as they contract, can pull on the retina and cause it to detach. The visual receptors (rods and cones) in the retina stop working when they are separated from the cells beneath them. Zones that have been detached show up as blanks in your field of vision.

What is macular edema?

Fluid leaking into the tissues of the retina causes swelling (edema). Leakage that settles in the macula area of the retina is called *diabetic macular edema* (DME) (Figure 4-4, in the color section). Edema that threatens the center of the macula is called *clinically significant macular edema* (CSME). The macula is responsible for detailed vision, so you may experience visual blur for both near and distant objects. Diabetic macular edema can sometimes cause you to be less sensitive to blue and yellow colors.

A person with uncontrolled type 2 diabetes is likely to develop macular edema. Because many people have uncontrolled type 2, macular edema accounts for most of the cases of vision loss from diabetes.

What puts you at risk for developing retinopathy?

How long you have had diabetes, your level of blood glucose control, and other medical conditions—such as hypertension, kidney disease, high cholesterol and other blood fat levels, and pregnancy—affect the development of diabetic retinopathy. People with high blood glucose levels are more likely to develop retinopathy.

If you have type 2 diabetes, you might have had some level of retinopathy when you were diagnosed, because most people with type 2 diabetes have it for awhile before they are diagnosed. (New diagnostic criteria have been introduced to help catch diabetes earlier than in the past.) You should have yearly eye examinations, because retinopathy can occur any time after diagnosis.

What are the symptoms of retinopathy?

All retinopathy begins as nonproliferative change. Depending on the severity and location, you may not have any symptoms or may complain of varying degrees of loss of central vision. Nonproliferative retinopathy causes vision loss when the macula becomes swollen or loses circulation.

Proliferative retinopathy begins to cause symptoms as the fragile new blood vessels break and leak into the vitreous gel. If blood flow is light, you may see floaters. If blood flow is heavy, you may only be able to distinguish between light and dark.

You may have serious, sight-threatening retinopathy even though you have no symptoms and vision can measure even better than 20/20 (normal vision). This is the reason annual eye examinations are so important. An exam to determine whether you need glasses or a change in your old prescription is not enough. You need a detailed examination of both the retina and the lens. Ophthalmologists and some optometrists are skilled in this exam. However, some optometrists do not do this full examination, so make sure that you ask.

Symptoms of changes in your retinas may include blurred or fluctuating vision, floating spots, distortion or warping of straight lines, or loss of vision. If you have symptoms, get an eye examination, even though you may not necessarily have serious problems. Remember, blurred vision could be caused by macular edema, but usually it results from natural aging or poor blood glucose control.

Distortion of straight lines can be a serious symptom. Many patients first notice such distortion while observing tiles or floor patterns with one eye closed. This distortion is often a sign of macular edema. Floating spots may be the result of age-related changes, but they may also indicate vitreous hemorrhage. A blockage of vision that is like a window shade being drawn across your field of view may indicate retinal detachment. With any symptom, play it safe, and have your eyes examined.

What happens at your eye examination?

Prevention and diagnosis of diabetic eye disease requires a thorough examination by an eye-care specialist experienced in managing diabetic eye disease. This examination should include measurement of your level of vision (visual acuity), evaluation of the movement of your eyes, refraction to determine your need for glasses, glaucoma screening, cataract evaluation, evaluation of changes in color perception or night vision, and dilation of your pupils to examine your retinas. Examination of the retina to detect retinopathy may require different techniques from those used in a routine eye examination. The eye-care specialist needs to be able to see your entire retina and vitreous gel.

The eye-care specialist may use a handheld ophthalmoscope, an indirect ophthalmoscope worn on his or her head, and/or the slit-lamp biomicroscope. The handheld, ophthalmoscope gives a magnified view of the optic nerve, macula, and blood vessels of the retina. The specialist can focus on the retina and detect the presence of hemorrhage, swelling, or the growth of new blood vessels.

The indirect ophthalmoscope, consisting of a head-light and handheld lenses, allows the eye-care specialist to examine the retina and determine areas of elevation. This is the best technique for identifying scar tissue on the surface of the retina and hemorrhages that may have settled by gravity to the bottom portion of the vitreous cavity.

You rest your chin on the slit-lamp biomicroscope while the eye-care specialist uses different lenses to examine the vitreous gel and retina. This instrument may help the specialist determine the presence of macular swelling. Occasionally, during this part of the examination, your eye may be anesthetized with drops, and a contact lens may be used.

Your pupil dilation and eye examination cause no harm to the retina. After the examination, you may have temporary dim vision or see various colors. Because of the pupil dilation, your vision may seem blurry for several hours, particularly for close-up work.

Are there other tests for diagnosing retinopathy?

Other diagnostic techniques that may be useful include fluorescein dye angiography and ultrasonography.

Fluorescein angiography

Fluorescein angiography is a technique in which pictures are taken of the retina while a fluorescent dye is flowing through its blood vessels. It requires an intravenous injection of the dye (usually in your arm) and a complex camera and lighting system. Details of the retinal circulation, including the smallest blood vessels, known as capillaries, can be evaluated by this technique. A series of up to 36 slides are taken to record the dye flow. Vessels that are healthy prevent the dye from leaking through the blood vessel walls. Vessels that are diseased allow the dye to leak. Accumulation of dye in the retina is a sign of edema. Leakage points that cause macular edema may be treated with focal laser surgery.

The fluorescein angiogram is a diagnostic test only; it is not a treatment. Following the test, you may notice your vision is temporarily blurred or dimmed, or you may see peculiar colors for a few moments. Vision rapidly returns to its pretest condition. You may notice a slight yellow or tan appearance to your skin and to the white of your eye lasting approximately 24 hours. The injected dye is cleared rapidly by way of the urinary system, giving a peculiar color to your urine. However, this dye can be safely used even in patients who have diabetic kidney disease, including patients who require dialysis.

You should be aware that the injection of any medicine or dye can be associated with complications, including allergic reactions. Fortunately, however, these are uncommon with fluorescein angiography. When the dye is first injected, you might feel a sensation of nausea that typically lasts only a few seconds. This is not an allergic reaction and should not prevent you from having future testing. The few patients who do suffer an allergic reaction to the fluorescein dye usually experience itching of their skin due to hives and rarely suffer a severe shocklike reaction. Patients who are allergic to the dye may, in fact, be able to undergo a future dye test with appropriate pre-operative medications and careful medical supervision.

Angiography is used to determine the extent of background retinopathy and particularly the points of leakage and areas that have lost circulation. These changes in the retina cannot be measured just by looking, and the angiogram is of great importance in helping to locate precise areas of leakage that require treatment. It also enables the physician to see whether there is impairment of the circulation of the macula, which is so vital to your sight. Angiography is not routinely used to detect proliferative retinopathy, except when hidden zones of blood vessel growth are suspected.

Ultrasonography

Using sound waves, ultrasound builds a picture of an area of the body that cannot be observed directly. It is a method for evaluating the back portion of the eye in people who have obstructions in the eye, such as advanced cataracts or hemorrhage in the vitreous gel. It may allow the physician to discover a retinal detachment or scar tissue on the surface of the retina. It does not provide a view of the retina itself, such as details of circulation abnormalities. Again, the ultrasound study is purely a method to diagnose and understand retinal anatomy and disease. Ultrasonography is particularly helpful in patients who have chronic vitreous hemorrhage and is often used before vitrectomy surgery (discussed below).

There are other tests to measure the thickness of the retina. These include optical coherence tomography, which uses ultrasound to measure the thickness of the retina and can give an indication of the degree of edema in a patient with nonproliferative (background) retinopathy. Such techniques have only recently been developed, and, although promising, their use is not yet widespread.

What is the treatment for nonproliferative retinopathy?

Blood glucose and blood pressure control are the crucial elements in treating diabetic eye disease. Treatment of nonproliferative retinopathy may involve the use of lasers to coagulate (seal) the places that are leaking or to make it easier for the retina to absorb the leakage. A fluorescein angiogram can be used to map areas that require treatment. Symptoms from background retinopathy may return as new zones of leakage develop. That is why you may require a series of treatments.

Nonproliferative retinopathy is classified as mild, moderate, severe, or very severe. It is important to determine the level of retinopathy because it indicates the risk of your eye progressing to sight-threatening proliferative retinopathy and determines how often you need to have eye examinations. Ask your eye doctor what level of retinopathy you have and to send a letter to your diabetes care provider. It is not enough to be told, "You have some eye changes, come back in a few months."

What is the treatment for proliferative retinopathy?

Proliferative retinopathy is treated with lasers, cryotherapy (freezing), and vitrectomy (removal of vitreous gel). The choice of which to use depends on several factors. Some patients have proliferative retinopathy only. Others have a combination of macular swelling and proliferation. Some patients may have associated hemorrhage, and others may have scar tissue pulling on the retina. Some patients may have cataracts obscuring the view of the retina. Occasionally, patients have new vessel growth on the iris as well, threatening to cause neovascular glaucoma. Each factor must be weighed by the ophthalmologist to determine the best course of management.

Laser treatment

The objective of treatment for proliferative retinopathy is to stop the abnormal blood vessels from growing and bleeding. Laser is the principal form of treatment used for this. The laser is used to destroy the ischemic areas of the retina that release growth factors and cause new blood vessels to grow. Destruction of these tissues causes the existing blood vessels to atrophy and prevents the growth of new blood vessels.

Laser also can be used to destroy abnormal blood vessels depending on their location (Figure 4-5, in the color section). If the blood vessels are on the surface of the retina away from the macula, they can be directly treated with the laser. This is called *focal laser treatment.* Focal laser surgery is usually performed in one treatment session and involves relatively few applications of the laser. Reevaluation is performed 2 or 3 months after treatment, and further treatment may be started if leaking and macular edema continue.

If the blood vessels are on the optic nerve surface, focal laser therapy could damage the optic nerve. Then the method is to scatter treatment throughout the retina to destroy the unhealthy zones. Treatment not only stops production of growth factors but also may increase the amount of oxygen getting to the remaining retina. The end result is to cut back the new blood vessels without using laser directly on the optic nerve. The scatter treatment is known as panretinal photocoagulation (Figure 4-6). It involves the application of approximately 1,200 to 1,800 laser beams in the midperipheral and peripheral (side) retina. The treatment is usually applied in two or three sessions. If all scatter laser surgery beams were applied in one session, it might cause excessive swelling in the retina and lead to macular edema, changes in vision, and, in extreme cases, angle-closure glaucoma.

Laser surgery is generally performed in the ophthalmologist's office as an outpatient procedure. The eye is anesthetized with an eyedrop similar to the drop used for glaucoma testing. A contact lens is placed on the eye, similar to the lens used for retinal examination by many eye doctors. This lens holds your eyelids open and focuses the laser light. In scatter laser photocoagulation, the laser applications are usually placed in rapid sequence, since less precise location is necessary. The ophthalmologist avoids large blood vessels, areas of hemorrhage, and the macula. Possible side effects of scatter laser photocoagulation include decreased night vision and some loss of peripheral vision. Sometimes laser treatments can alter color vision (Table 4-1). Focal laser surgery involves fewer laser applications (usually fewer than 100), but the applications are placed much more precisely. Consequently, it will take more time between applications as the ophthalmologist focuses the laser in precise position.

Laser treatment is modified for patients who also have nonproliferative retinopathy with macular edema, hemorrhage, scar tissue on the retina, or cataract. For patients who do not have macular edema, focal or panretinal scatter treatment can be done in one or more sessions. The physician usually treats the lower portion of the retina first, so that any bleeding would be likely to settle in the region of the retina that has already been treated. This would allow the physician to see clearly to complete the treatment to the top portion of the retina. Depending on the degree of treatment required, one or more sessions may be necessary.

For patients who also have macular edema, it is desirable to treat the swelling first and then do the panretinal treatment for the proliferative retinopathy. The goal is to reduce the swelling because panretinal treatment may also cause swelling. In this instance, points of leakage surrounding the macula get focal treatment. Then, in multiple sessions, panretinal scatter treatment can be done to the overgrowth of blood vessels.

In patients who have preexisting scar tissue on the retina, the ophthalmologist may need multiple sessions to avoid the areas of scar tissue and prevent contracting them further.

Patients with a cataract may present a challenge because the cataract may prevent examination of the retina and block the laser from reaching the retina.

Table 4-1. Possible Side Effects and Complications of Laser Treatment

Side effects

- Temporary blurring of vision
- Decreased peripheral vision
- Diminished night vision
- Reduced near-focusing ability
- Unequal pupil size
- Light sensitivity

Complications

- Corneal burn
- Lenticular burn
- Macular burn
- Pain
- Macular edema
- Retinal traction involving the macula
- Angle-closure glaucoma
- Vitreous hemorrhage

The Uncomplicated Guide to Diabetes Complications

Lasers that produce red wavelengths of light may be particularly helpful in patients who have a cataract because they are transmitted through the cataract better. Occasionally, it is necessary to do cataract surgery first to be able to see and treat the retina. However, physicians generally prefer to treat the retina before doing cataract surgery and then evaluate the eye once again after the cataract has been removed.

For patients who also have a vitreous hemorrhage, laser treatment may be difficult to do. Patients with such hemorrhages are advised to sleep with the head of the bed elevated and to avoid bending with their head below the heart so that gravity will help the hemorrhage to settle in the lower portion of the eye. Not exercising may also help the hemorrhage to settle and allow the ophthalmologist to examine and treat the upper portions of the retina. As the hemorrhage settles, more of the retina becomes visible, and the panretinal treatment can be completed. The image you see is reversed by the eye, so if you have a hemorrhage that settles in the bottom of your eye, you will see the floating debris at the top of your field of vision.

Cryotherapy

Cryotherapy (freezing) is sometimes used for the management of proliferative retinopathy. Cryotherapy allows treatment of the far edges of the retina that can't be reached by laser. Cryotherapy is useful in patients who previously have had complete laser treatment but still have neovascularization (new blood vessel growth) and bleeding. Cryotherapy may also be useful in individuals who have hemorrhage that prevents the completion of the laser treatment.

Vitrectomy

For the few patients who have chronic vitreous hemorrhage that does not go away or for patients with hemorrhages in both eyes who cannot carry out their normal daily functions such as eating, dressing, or taking medications, vitrectomy surgery may be indicated (Figures 4-7a, 4-7b, in the color section). A hemorrhage on the surface of the retina that blocks the macula is often a reason for vitrectomy surgery because such hemorrhages tend to go away slowly and may result in the formation of scar tissue that covers the macula and pulls on the retina.

What happens in laser surgery?

Physicians vary in the methods they use to treat the retina, and the methods described below are just common examples.

Lasers create thin beams of light of differing wavelengths or colors. Ophthalmic lasers creating green, red, yellow, or infrared wavelengths can be used to clot leaking blood vessels, destroy zones of overgrown blood vessels, or destroy zones of ischemic retina. The laser light penetrates the eye; travels through the aqueous, lens, and vitreous; and is absorbed in the deepest layers of the retina, where the light energy is converted to heat. The heat seals the surrounding area, which heals as a laser scar.

Different wavelengths of light may serve useful purposes. For instance, red wavelengths penetrate blood in the vitreous or a cataract better than green wavelengths. The photoreceptors (rods and cones) in the areas that are treated are destroyed by the treatment, and thus laser scars are typically blank spots in the field of vision. These blank spots generally don't bother you because they are tiny, are located away from the central area responsible for detail vision, or involve areas with poor circulation (ischemia) that have already stopped working.

Anesthesia

The need for anesthesia varies. It is important for you to remain still during treatment. Most patients do this by staring at a target with the eye that is not being treated while the other eye is being treated. If you cannot remain immobile or if anesthetic drops in your eyes are not enough, then a local anesthesia by injection into the tissues surrounding the eye is used. Some cases require treatment extraordinarily close to the center of the macula, the most visually sensitive zone of the retina. In these cases, the physician may choose to immobilize your eye by injecting a local anesthetic into the tissues around the eye. As a rule, laser treatment causes little discomfort. However, depending on the amount of treatment required or depending on specific regions of the retina that need treatment, some patients may experience localized discomfort during treatment or a posttreatment headache.

Laser surgery procedure

Laser can be administered either through a slit lamp or through an indirect ophthalmoscope. At the slit lamp, you are seated and rest your chin and forehead in a stabilizing device. A contact lens is put in position on the surface of your cornea, and the physician can see your retina. The physician may project photographic images of the retina or of the fluorescein angiogram to use as a map to locate the points that require treatment. The physician will choose the appropriate wavelength of light for your retina. The laser typically emits a very-low-power aiming beam that the physician can direct to the point needing treatment. When the laser is fired, that aiming beam becomes intensified, and the resulting laser light hits the target. The physician can immediately see the point that is treated and check the result. The physician can use different-sized laser beams to treat abnormalities of differing sizes in the retina. Often, leaky points may be treated with very small spots of laser, but scatter panretinal treatment may be done with larger laser spots. The physician can alter the laser not only in the size of the beam but also in its duration and power. The physician may use a variety of contact lenses on you to see your entire retina.

Indirect ophthalmoscope laser treatment is particularly good for treatment to the far edge of the retina. Commonly, this requires injection of a local anesthetic to eliminate motion of the eye and to prevent discomfort during treatment. This technique is more commonly employed for panretinal scatter photocoagulation treatment.

Cryotherapy procedure

Cryotherapy of the retina is typically performed with you lying on your back. The surface of the eye is anesthetized, creating a regional block anesthesia. Your eyelids are separated with a device known as a speculum to hold them in an open position. The physician examines your retina using the indirect ophthalmoscope to see the far edge of the retina. Cryotherapy is applied with a probe connected to a cold source. The cryoprobe can be placed on the surface of the eye. When the probe is properly located, the freezing process can begin. The tip of the probe rapidly reaches a very low temperature and creates an actual freeze that extends from the soft external tissues through the wall of the eye until it reaches the retina. The physician can see the freeze directly. Multiple points of the retina can be treated in this fashion.

Vitrectomy procedure

Vitrectomy is a microsurgical procedure for removal of the core of the vitreous gel, which may be extremely cloudy or may be pulling on the retina in the case of diabetic retinopathy, and replacing it with a clear fluid similar to the fluid in the eye.

Vitrectomy is performed in a darkened operating room. It requires anesthetic, either a local regional anesthetic or general anesthesia. General anesthesia may be preferred if you will require a more prolonged surgical procedure or if you are anxious and unable to tolerate being awake during surgery.

Once the anesthesia has taken effect, the surgeon makes small incisions to allow access to the sclera, or wall, of your eye. Typically, three very small openings are made through the wall of the eye into the vitreous cavity. One opening allows new clear fluids to flow in. This maintains the correct pressure within the eye and replaces the darkened vitreous fluid that may be removed in the course of surgery. The other two openings are used by the surgeon, one to illuminate and the other to manipulate the tissues of your eye. An operating microscope is positioned over your eye, and with various contact lenses, the surgeon can see the vitreous cavity, its contents, and the underlying retinal tissue.

The initial step is to clear the vitreous cavity. In patients who have a hemorrhage, the vitreous often is partially or completely filled with blood. This blood is removed, and the cavity is filled with clear fluid. Patients who have a clear vitreous but underlying scar tissue or retinal detachment also undergo removal of the vitreous gel and replacement of it with clear fluid. This allows the surgeon to pass the required instruments safely to the retinal surface without snagging or pulling on the vitreous gel.

Once the vitreous cavity has been cleared, surgery on the surface of the retina can be done. This may include vacuuming blood from the surface. Patients often have scar tissue and blood vessels extending from the retina up into the vitreous cavity. These scars can be cut free from the retina and treated directly to seal their blood vessels. Scarring that has caused retinal detachment can be removed, and the detached retina will gradually settle back into its normal position.

The surgeon can insert a probe through the vitreous to deliver laser treatment to the retina at the completion of the surgery. In some instances, patients will have underlying tears or holes in the retina. Often, these are managed with laser treatment combined with a gas bubble. A gas bubble holds the margins of the retinal tear against the back wall of the eye until the laser treatment can create a secure seal.

Various gases are used to hold the retina in place postoperatively until healing is complete. Some gases last only a few days, and others last several months. While gas is in the eye, you will notice markedly reduced vision. As the gas is absorbed, you frequently will notice a portion of your vision is blocked by the gas bubble, but the area not covered by the gas has normal vision. The gas bubble will separate into multiple tiny bubbles and then be absorbed. As absorption takes place, the vitreous cavity is naturally refilled by the eye's normal production of aqueous fluid. After vitrectomy, with or without gas injection, the vitreous cavity is refilled by the naturally occurring aqueous fluid. Before your surgery, the aqueous filled only a small portion of the eye, but now it fills the vitreous cavity as well as the front portion of the eye. The vitreous is not replaced, and its absence is not damaging to the eye.

Generally, vitrectomy surgery has a lasting beneficial effect for patients with proliferative retinopathy. Occasionally, patients have a small persistent hemorrhage after surgery that often clears on its own. Other patients may rebleed, but again this usually clears spontaneously. A few patients will have repetitive bleeding or regrowth of scar tissue that requires repeat vitrectomy, but this is uncommon. Once your retinopathy has been stabilized by vitrectomy, it typically remains stable for the rest of your life. It is uncommon for vitrectomy patients to have recurrent proliferation later in life.

Vitrectomy surgery, like any other surgical intervention, has potential complications. Sight-threatening complications are rare. However, it is common for cataracts to form in eyes that have had vitrectomy. You should be aware that an additional surgical procedure, namely cataract surgery, may be required in an eye that has had successful vitrectomy.

What do you need to do after having treatment for retinopathy?

The most important thing you can do after any kind of treatment for retinopathy is to control your blood glucose and blood pressure levels.

Laser

After laser treatment, you may not need any eye medication. Some patients need a brief course of eye drops to reduce inflammation. If you have postoperative pain, it can easily be treated with oral pain relievers. If only anesthetic drops were used, you may not require a patch on your eye. However, if a regional anesthetic was used, the eye may be patched until the anesthesia wears off and the eye is working normally.

Cryotherapy

After treatment, the outer surface of the eye is often swollen. It may appear red for 1–2 weeks. You may be treated with eyedrops for inflammation. You may feel a moderate degree of discomfort, depending on the amount of treatment you need. Oral pain medications can usually make you feel better. Narcotics are rarely needed. Cryotherapy is generally accomplished as an outpatient procedure and only occasionally requires hospitalization.

Vitrectomy

Vitrectomy may be either an inpatient or an outpatient procedure. A variety of medications may be used after surgery, including drops to dilate the pupil, inhibit infection, and reduce inflammation. Depending on the extent of the surgery, you may require pain medication immediately by injection, but more commonly, you will be comfortable using oral pain medications.

Typically, you will have swelling and redness of the tissues of the eye. The swelling and redness will go away over a 3-week period. At that time, you can resume wearing contact lenses, if you have them.

During the postoperative period, you may be asked to maintain certain head positions. You may have a small amount of hemorrhage in the eye. To help clear the hemorrhage, you will be asked to sleep with the head of the bed elevated and to avoid bending.

If a gas bubble was placed in the vitreous cavity, you may be asked to position yourself to allow the gas bubble to press against treated areas of the retina until the gas is absorbed and replaced by the aqueous fluid of the eye. **You should not fly in any aircraft until the bubble is gone.** If you must have another general anesthetic during the postoperative period, be sure to tell your physician about the gas in your eye. Such anesthesia can be done safely, but the anesthesiologist must know that the gas is present in the vitreous cavity of your eye. Depending on your vision in the other eye and requirements for transportation or work, you may need a period of inactivity, including a leave of absence from work.

How does vision change after treatment for retinopathy?

Patients treated for macular swelling occasionally notice tiny blank spots in their field of vision, but these usually are not troublesome. After scatter panretinal treatment, some patients may notice a decrease in night vision, color vision, or peripheral vision. Most patients are unaware of such changes because these are the symptoms that gradually developed with the onset of retinopathy. A temporary decrease in central vision is common, and some patients may experience a permanent slight reduction in vision. Temporary glare and difficulty focusing on near objects is a common occurrence after scatter treatment but generally goes away over several weeks.

It is not possible to predict how your vision will be improved after laser treatment or vitrectomy. As described in this chapter, there are many causes for loss of vision, and you may have several of them. For instance, treating macular swelling or neovascular tissue will not alter the age-related development of cataracts. Removal of hemorrhage by vitrectomy will clear the path for light to reach the retina, but the health of the underlying retina can't be determined until surgery is done.

The unknown and the fear that laser or surgery may harm vision often make a patient decide to delay therapy. Although there are potential risks in any form of treatment, the risks of untreated retinopathy generally greatly outweigh the risk of treatment. Without treatment, diabetic retinopathy is usually progressive and sight threatening. Treatment with laser and vitrectomy have been proven to benefit vision. Prompt diagnosis of retinopathy and appropriate treatment are the key elements for your successful visual outcome.

The best time for laser surgery is before you lose any vision. Detecting retinopathy just as it reaches a treatable stage is the most important factor in preventing visual loss from this disease.

How effective are these treatments for retinopathy?

Four nationwide clinical trials—the Diabetic Retinopathy Study (DRS), the Early Treatment Diabetic Retinopathy Study (ETDRS), the Diabetic Retinopathy Vitrectomy Study (DRVS), and the Diabetes Control and Complications Trial (DCCT)—set the standards for diagnosing and treating diabetic eye disease. These studies show that scatter laser surgery for proliferative retinopathy and focal laser surgery for macular edema significantly reduce your risk of vision loss. For example, a person with proliferative retinopathy who does not get treatment has a 60% risk of severe vision loss over 5 years. Laser surgery reduces this risk to less than 5%.

What else can you do to prevent or control retinopathy?

We know from the DCCT that intensive control of blood sugar levels in people with type 1 diabetes significantly reduces the risk of onset of any retinopathy, slows the progression of retinopathy once it is present, and reduces the need for laser surgery. Studies of people with type 2 diabetes on tight control demonstrate that they get the same benefits. Therefore, you would be wise to try to keep your blood sugar levels as close to normal as possible. See your physician for the targets that are right for you.

What about other eye changes caused by diabetes?

All structures of the eye can be affected by diabetes (Table 4-2). Some of the effects are not sight-threatening but are frustrating and may interfere with daily tasks such as reading and driving. Other effects may reflect disease in other organs, such as the kidneys. In some instances, visual changes may be attributed to diabetes when they are actually not related to diabetes at all.

Why is your vision blurred or fluctuating?

You can have fluctuations in vision because of uncontrolled blood glucose levels without permanent changes to the eye. Frequently, higher levels of blood glucose can cause you to become more near-sighted. Your distance vision may become blurred, while near vision may actually seem clearer. Some people may even find they don't need reading glasses. Such changes in vision may be temporary.

What are cataracts?

A cataract is any cloudiness in the lens of the eye. Some cataracts have no effect on your vision, but cataracts that interfere with vision need to be treated. Cataracts tend to develop at a younger age and progress more rapidly in people with diabetes. Cataracts are generally viewed as a condition affecting people 60 years of age or older, and most cataracts tend to progress gradually. It is not unusual, however, for people with diabetes to develop cataracts in their 30s or 40s, and the progression of the cataract can be dramatic. Cataracts specifically related to diabetes are sometimes caused by very poorly controlled blood glucose levels. Sometimes, adolescents or adults with new-onset diabetes that is poorly controlled develop diabetic cataracts, but these cataracts are relatively rare.

What are the symptoms of cataracts?

Symptoms of cataracts may include a dulling of vision, decreased reading vision, higher reading light requirements, or difficulty driving. Sometimes, cataracts cause car headlights to have a star-burst or sparkler effect.

What is the treatment for cataracts?

When cataracts interfere enough with vision to prevent you from performing necessary tasks of daily living, surgery may be indicated. Cataract surgery today is generally performed as an outpatient procedure. In most cases, the lens is surgically removed from the eye. A plastic lens, whose power and characteristics are determined in preoperative evaluations, is then implanted in the eye. Generally, the surgeon will intentionally leave the posterior membrane, or lens capsule, in place in the eye. This capsule continues to separate the two sections of the eye.

Cataract surgery itself is not performed with a laser; however, with time, the lens capsule may become cloudy, much like an original cataract. This condition is frequently referred to as an aftercataract. Aftercataracts are routinely treated with a laser, which opens a permanent clear hole in the cloudy lens capsule. The laser used for this treatment is different from the lasers used to treat diabetic retinopathy.

After cataract surgery, glasses are usually still required for best vision—for reading, for distance, or for both. The lens implant fixes the focus of the eye for only one distance, but glasses allow the flexibility of focusing at different distances.

What is glaucoma?

As a person with diabetes, you are twice as likely to develop glaucoma as someone without diabetes. Glaucoma is a condition in which the pressure inside the eye (known as intraocular pressure) causes damage to the optic nerve. Generally, increased pressure causes damage.

Table 4-2. Diabetic Effects on the Eye and Vision

Structure/ Function	Complication	Management
Refraction/focus	• Fluctuating vision • Refractive error • Early presbyopia • Reduced accommodation	• Rule out nondiabetes causes • Control blood glucose levels • Eyeglass prescription • Low vision/vision rehabilitation
Intraocular pressure (IOP)	• Open-angle glaucoma • Narrow-angle glaucoma • Neovascular glaucoma	• Monitor IOP • Treat glaucoma as indicated • Scatter laser photocoagulation or photocoagulation for neovascular glaucoma
Extraocular muscles	• Mononeuropathy	• Rule out nondiabetes causes • Temporary spectacle prisms to relieve diplopia • Temporary eye patching to relieve diplopia • Neurologist consultation
Cornea	• Reduced corneal sensitivity • Recurrent corneal abrasion • Corneal ulceration • Delayed corneal healing	• Tear substitutes/eyedrops • Infection control • Safety glasses • Careful contact lens evaluation and monitoring
Iris	• Rubeosis iridis	• Evaluation of filtration angle • Comprehensive fundus evaluation • Scatter laser photocoagulation as indicated • Control of IOP
Lens	• Cataract	• Monitor cataract progression and level of retinopathy • Cataract surgery and intraocular lens implant as indicated
Retina	• Diabetic retinopathy • Diabetic macular edema	• Monitor level of retinopathy • Focal laser treatment or scatter laser treatment as indicated

* Eye complications should be managed by ophthalmologists or optometrists trained and experienced in treating diabetic eye disease. Patient education is an important part of management of all complications.

The eye constantly produces and drains a fluid known as the aqueous. This fluid is not a component of our tears and does not come to the outer surface of the eye. The balance of production and drainage determines the pressure in the eye (see Figure 4-1).

The same loss of blood supply that causes new blood vessels to grow on the retina also causes them to grow across the drainage network and block the fluid from leaving the eye. The eye keeps on making fluid but cannot drain it. The eye is rigid and not elastic; it does not enlarge. Therefore, the pressure inside the eye increases and eventually damages the optic nerve.

There are many types of glaucoma. The most common form of glaucoma is open-angle glaucoma. It is caused by obstruction of the drainage network, which is also called the filtration angle. Usually, open-angle glaucoma causes no symptoms or changes in vision until damage is advanced. Damage usually occurs over a prolonged period and progresses gradually.

In angle-closure glaucoma, fluid can't drain because the filtration angle is too narrow. Angle closure can occur spontaneously or can even be caused by dilation of the pupils, which is a normal part of a comprehensive eye examination. A comprehensive eye examination, however, can usually determine whether an eye is prone to angle closure, and treatment can prevent angle-closure attacks. A person with angle-closure glaucoma may experience excruciating pain in the eye and rapid decrease in vision, although pain may be caused by other problems such as foreign bodies in the eye or scratches on the cornea. If angle closure is not complete, a person may have angle-closure attacks, which may result in the appearance of haloes around lights. Diabetes does not pose a greater risk for angle-closure glaucoma.

Another type of glaucoma is neovascular glaucoma. In neovascular glaucoma, new blood vessels grow on the surface of the iris and eventually reach and block the filtration angle. Diabetes can be a risk factor for neovascular glaucoma, particularly if proliferative diabetic retinopathy is present. There may be no symptoms, or there may be symptoms similar to those of angle-closure glaucoma.

What is the treatment for glaucoma?

Treatment for glaucoma depends on the type of glaucoma. Open-angle glaucoma is generally treated with eyedrops initially. Laser treatments to the filtration angle are sometimes indicated if the glaucoma does not respond to eyedrops or other medications.

Management of angle-closure glaucoma is to prevent angle closure. Laser treatments can be used to create a small hole in the iris of the eye, allowing fluid to pass from one section of the eye to the other. Such treatment, called a laser iridotomy, usually cures and prevents angle-closure glaucoma, although careful follow-up evaluations are needed. Angle-closure glaucoma is an emergency and may be treated with eyedrops, laser therapy, and/or surgery.

Neovascular glaucoma is usually treated with laser surgery to the retina, because the new vessels grow as the result of retinal dysfunction. Eyedrops or laser treatment to the vessels themselves may be necessary if the glaucoma does not respond to laser treatment of the retina. Once again, it is crucial that the patient has follow-up visits to the eye-care specialist during the active stages of these conditions.

Can diabetes affect the optic nerve in other ways?

Diabetes can damage blood vessels and restrict the blood flow through them. The optic nerve is damaged whenever it does not receive its own blood supply. Initially, it swells. It may then recover, but some atrophy often follows. The atrophy, which consists of a loss of nerve fibers, is permanent and may result in loss of a portion of your field of vision or both the peripheral field and central vision.

A loss of blood supply to the visual nerve pathways in the brain can also damage your vision. This loss of circulation is commonly called a stroke and is known as a cerebrovascular accident (CVA) (see chapter 7). Sometimes a clot may block a blood vessel only briefly and then move on. This will cause a temporary loss of some part or all of your vision that clears up on its own. Bring these symptoms to the attention of your doctor to determine the cause and location of the obstruction and to prevent it from happening again.

What happens when you have double vision?

Diabetes can sometimes result in double vision (diplopia). The position of the human eye is controlled by six muscles that surround the eye. Each eye has its own muscles and nerve supply, and the movements of both eyes are coordinated so that they maintain focus simultaneously on a given visual target. Diabetes can do damage to both blood vessels and nerves. If one nerve is impaired by lack of blood supply, the muscle cannot move the eye, and the coordination is disrupted. The two eyes are focused on two different targets, and the brain gets two distinct images, causing double vision.

Decreased blood supply to the nerves that activate the muscles of the eye can cause a full or partial paralysis of the eye muscles supplied by the nerve. This is called mononeuropathy. Symptoms of mononeuropathy include sudden onset of double vision, drooping of the eyelid, and sometimes pain over the affected eye. Treatment of this condition can be to patch either eye to eliminate one of the two images or to use an optical device called a prism in a spectacle lens in an attempt to align the two eyes. In general, the nerve regains its function over several months, and the eyes again track together. Rarely, surgery on the muscle is required to realign the eyes so they can maintain a single image.

Double vision may be the first sign of serious or life-threatening conditions. Immediate eye examination and careful evaluation by a doctor familiar with diabetic eye disease is critical.

Does physical activity affect retinopathy?

Regular exercise is an important element of blood glucose control. In general, physical activity and exercise do not affect vision in cases of macular edema or nonproliferative retinopathy. In cases of active proliferative retinopathy, however—particularly if vitreous hemorrhage, fibrous tissue, or significant new vessel growth is present—some types of physical activity might be harmful. Exertion may cause those new blood vessels to rupture, resulting in vitreous hemorrhage. Also, exertion may lead to retinal detachment if significant retinal traction is present. Contact sports that involve jarring, high-impact aerobics, and lifting free weights might cause you problems. Although retinopathy does not interfere with most forms of exercise and activity, your comprehensive eye examination will help you and your physician determine the best level of exercise.

What can you do to reduce your risk of vision loss?

You need to take an active role in your own eye care. There are very effective ways to reduce your risk of diabetic retinopathy. The best way to prevent severe diabetic retinopathy is to control your blood glucose and blood pressure levels. Generally, you should also

- maintain a regular eye examination schedule as determined by your eye doctor (Table 4-3)
- maintain as good control of other medical conditions as possible, especially kidney disease, blood cholesterol, and triglycerides

Your recommended eye examination schedule includes

- Initial examination within 3–5 years of diagnosis for people 10 years or older, and at least annual examination thereafter for type 1 diabetes
- examination at diagnosis of type 2 diabetes, and at least annual examination thereafter
- examination before planned pregnancy or early in the first trimester of any pregnancy and close follow-up throughout pregnancy

More frequent examination may be necessary based on the level of retinopathy and the presence of other medical conditions.

In conclusion

With rigorous and lifelong eye examinations, more than 98% of legal blindness from diabetic retinopathy can be prevented. Becoming educated and involved in your own health care, maintaining good blood glucose and blood pressure control, and having routine eye examinations can dramatically reduce the tragic burden of vision loss from diabetes.

This chapter was written by M. Gilbert Grand, MD; Lloyd Paul Aiello, MD, PhD; Jerry D. Cavallerano, OD, PhD; and Mami A. Iwamoto, MD.

Table 4-3. Suggested Frequency of Eye Examinations

Type of Diabetes	Recommended 1st Examination	Routine Minimal Follow-Up
Type 1	For people 10 yrs or older 3–5 years after onset	Yearly
Type 2	On diagnosis	Yearly
During Pregnancy	• Before conception for counseling • Early in 1st trimester	• Each trimester • More frequently as indicated • 3–6 months postpartum

5

Heart Disease

Introduction

Cardiovascular disease and stroke are the most common causes of death in the U.S.adult population. They cause 900,000 deaths annually, or more than 42% of all deaths in the U.S. About 56 million Americans have some form of heart disease—heart attack, stroke, congenital heart defects, hypertension, or obstruction of the arteries. Adults with diabetes are three times more likely to die of cardiovascular disease than the general population. Diabetes puts you at serious risk for several forms of heart and vascular disease—coronary artery disease, heart attack, and sudden death (Table 5-1). Keeping your blood sugar as close to normal as possible can decrease the likelihood of your having cardiovascular complications.

What is coronary artery disease?

Coronary artery disease (CAD) is an illness in which some of your heart muscle does not receive sufficient blood, oxygen, and nutrients to meet its needs because of partial or complete blockage of the coronary blood vessels, which supply the heart. The most common cause of CAD is atherosclerosis, or hardening of the arteries. In

Table 5-1. Forms of Cardiovascular Disease Associated with Diabetes

- Coronary artery disease
  - Angina
  - Heart attack
  - Sudden death
- Congestive heart failure
  - Diabetic cardiomyopathy
  - Coronary artery disease
  - Ischemic cardiomyopathy
- Hypertension
- Peripheral vascular disease
- Anatomic dysfunction

this disease, cholesterol builds up in the walls of the coronary vessels gradually over many years. The process is complex. There is usually some initial damage to the lining of the major arteries of the heart. Common causes of this injury include hypertension, diabetes, cigarette smoking, and high blood cholesterol levels. The body's response to this injury encourages scavenger cells (macrophages) to enter the damaged areas to repair the injury. However, macrophages, and substances they produce, contribute to blocking the vessels. After many cycles of injury and attempted repair, deposits of cholesterol and scar tissue can build up and block the vessel partially or completely.

What puts you at risk for developing CAD?

Diabetes, a family history of CAD, hypertension, smoking, high cholesterol, advancing age, sedentary lifestyle, high triglycerides, and obesity are all risk factors for CAD. The higher your blood cholesterol level, the higher your risk of CAD. Cholesterol is carried in the blood in several forms, including low-density lipoprotein (LDL) and high-density lipoprotein (HDL) cholesterol. There is a direct relationship between LDL ("bad") cholesterol and the risk of CAD—the risk increases as LDL increases. However, increasing levels of HDL ("good") cholesterol protects against your risk of developing CAD. (See chapter 6 for more on cholesterol.)

Years of cigarette smoking increase your risk of developing CAD. The good news is that quitting helps. The risk from smoking decreases when you have not smoked for 5 years.

People with impaired glucose tolerance (IGT) are at higher risk for developing angina and heart attack than people with normal glucose tolerance, and people with diabetes are at an even higher risk. Most physicians believe that people whose diabetes is poorly controlled are at higher risk for CAD and heart attack than those whose diabetes is tightly controlled. There is also a direct relationship between how long you have had diabetes and the likelihood of developing CAD. A person who has had diabetes for 15–20 years is 10 times as likely to develop CAD as people in the general population.

What are the symptoms of CAD?

When 50–75% of a blood vessel is blocked, the limited blood flow can cause you to experience symptoms. Generally, the symptoms occur first with exercise, because the heart requires more fuel when heart rate and blood pressure increase. The most common symptom is pain (angina) or pressure in the chest (Table 5-2); however, the symptoms can vary. The pain usually comes on gradually over a period of 30 seconds to several minutes. It may become more severe, or it may remain mild and then go

Table 5-2. Symptoms of Coronary Artery Disease

- Chest pain/pressure
  - Under the breast bone, in the left arm, shoulder, neck, or jaw
  - Pressure (or tightness)
  - Gradual onset (over 30 seconds to minutes)
  - Gradual resolution
  - Related to physical or emotional stress
- Shortness of breath
  - Usually associated with chest pain or physical or emotional stress
- Nausea
  - Usually associated with chest pain or shortness of breath and physical or emotional stress
- Palpitation, Fainting, Sudden death
  - Related to irregular heartbeat caused by insufficient blood flow to the heart muscle

away. The pain may move to the left arm, shoulder, armpit, or left side of the neck or jaw. Typically, the discomfort comes on with exercise and is relieved by rest. However, the pain can come on at rest, or even awaken you from sleep. The pain may also begin during emotional stress, such as an argument at work or at home.

You may not have pain or pressure in the chest. Some people complain mainly of nausea or discomfort in the upper abdomen, often mistaken for heartburn. Sometimes these symptoms are relieved by belching or by taking antacids, which can be confusing for both you and your physician. These are also symptoms of gastroparesis, gallbladder disease, and other gastrointestinal disturbances—diseases that people with diabetes are more likely to have (see chapter 13). Also, some people with diabetes have nerve damage and are unable to feel the discomfort that would normally be present (sensory cardiac neuropathy), just as some people develop foot ulcers in part because of their inability to feel injuries to their feet (see chapters 3 and 11). The only symptoms may be caused by the part of the heart muscle that is not receiving sufficient blood. You may be short of breath because your heart cannot pump blood out into the body, so the blood backs up into the lungs. Sometimes patients become weak because the brain is not getting the blood and oxygen it needs. A heart that is receiving insufficient blood may beat rapidly or irregularly.

When symptoms last only 2–15 minutes and do not occur more frequently or at lower levels of exercise, and heart tests show no evidence of permanent damage, you have *stable angina.* When the symptoms abruptly get worse or begin occurring at rest, the pattern is called *unstable angina,* a warning sign of serious heart trouble. Sometimes the progressive nature of the symptoms can precede a heart attack (myocardial infarction).

How does autonomic neuropathy affect your cardiovascular system?

Autonomic nerves control your heart rate and blood pressure. In people who do not have neuropathy, blood pressure and heart rate change slightly throughout the day in response to position (lying, sitting, and standing), stress, exercise, breathing patterns, and sleep. If the nerves to the heart and blood vessels are damaged by diabetes, the blood pressure and heart rate may respond more slowly to these factors.

If the nerves that regulate your blood pressure are damaged, the blood pressure can drop quickly when you stand up and not return to a normal level as quickly as it did before the nerves were damaged. You can feel lightheaded and dizzy, see black spots, or even pass out. This is called *orthostatic hypotension* (see chapter 12).

If the nerves that control heart rate are affected, the heart rate tends to be fast and does not change as quickly in response to breathing patterns, exercise, stress, or sleep. This is diagnosed by measuring the rise and fall of your heart rate as you breathe deeply or by a Valsalva maneuver (when you bear down as hard as you can). An electrocardiogram (ECG) may be used to do this. It is a serious complication because it may increase your risk for an irregular heartbeat and prevent the pain or other warning symptoms of a heart attack.

Another cardiac problem caused by autonomic neuropathy is the absence of heart pain (angina). A patient may have a so-called silent heart attack, which is a heart attack without pain. Thus, one explanation for diabetes that suddenly gets out of control may be the stress of a heart attack even though there is no chest pain (see chapter 12).

How can your doctor diagnose CAD?

CAD may be diagnosed in several ways. Initially, the symptoms alert you and your health care provider to the possibility that you have it. The more classic your symptoms (location, character, relationship to exercise, etc.) and the greater your number of risk factors, the more likely that you actually have CAD. At this point, any of several diagnostic tests can be used to confirm the diagnosis.

An ECG performed at rest can help the physician diagnose a heart attack that occurred sometime in the past (or one that is occurring at the time of the ECG). As many as one-third of all heart attacks are clinically silent—that is, you don't notice any symptoms at the time of the heart attack—but an ECG performed at a later date indicates what happened. However, coronary blockages that have not yet caused a heart attack may not show up on a resting ECG.

Stress testing is performed by examining you and obtaining ECGs before, during, and after exercise on a treadmill or exercise bicycle. The level of exercise is increased in steps until you develop symptoms that cause you to stop, you become fatigued, the ECG becomes very abnormal, or you reach a predetermined maximum heart rate. Stress testing can be performed with just an ECG, a cardiac ultrasound test, or scanning of radioactive tracers to determine whether coronary blood flow abnormalities are present. When ultrasound and radioactive tracers are used, they are monitored with the ECG. When someone who has partially or completely blocked coronary arteries exercises, some of the heart muscle may not receive sufficient blood. This condition can result in characteristic changes in the ECG. The stress ECG is only moderately accurate for diagnosing CAD. About 70% of patients with significant blockage who exercise (increasing heart rates to more than 85% of maximum heart rate for their age) will have a positive test. However, only about 70% of these patients will actually have obstructions in their coronary arteries. Therefore, most people have both exercise stress testing and a heart imaging test.

When an echocardiogram (heart ultrasound) is performed before and immediately after exercise, the accuracy of the test improves substantially. If blockages are present, the area with limited blood flow moves abnormally when you exercise, and the cardiologist can make a more accurate assessment of the extent and severity of the problem.

Some stress tests are performed with nuclear imaging before and after exercise. This procedure helps to determine the level of blood flow to different parts of the heart, so the doctor can assess how many and how large the obstructions are. The echo and nuclear stress tests detect significantly abnormal coronary arteries in about 90% of people tested. Only 90% of these people actually have significantly obstructed vessels. The more severe the CAD is, the more likely the tests will show it.

What if you cannot exercise?

Many people with suspected CAD cannot exercise because they have another disease such as asthma, emphysema, peripheral vascular disease with claudication (aching in the legs during exercise), or amputation. For these people, cardiologists use chemical stress tests. In these tests, the echocardiogram or nuclear imaging is done before and after stress with drugs such as dobutamine (which increases the work of the heart), or adenosine or dipyridamole (which expand the arteries of the heart). The accuracy of stress testing using drugs is similar to that of tests using exercise.

What happens when your test is positive?

If your stress test is positive, your doctor may start you on oral medications to reduce symptoms, slow the progression of CAD, and extend your life. Or you may be scheduled for *cardiac catheterization* and *coronary angiography*. In this procedure, the cardiologist examines your heart using a plastic catheter (tube) inserted into an artery (usually in the groin) after you've been given a local anesthetic. The catheters are threaded up the major vessels into the chest so that blood pressures can be checked in the different chambers of the heart. X-ray dye can flow through the tubes into your heart and heart arteries so that the physician can observe the overall function of your heart, whether some walls are moving normally, and whether there are large obstructions in the arteries. Depending on the results, you may not need special treatment (your stress test had a false positive result). Otherwise, you may need oral or topical medicines for angina, a procedure to open the artery mechanically (*angioplasty*) or heart surgery to bypass the obstructions. These decisions are complex and depend on your anatomy, the number and severity of blockages, their locations, the size of the openings in the vessels, and the pump function of your heart.

What medications should you take for CAD?

Nitroglycerin

Several classes of medication are available if your physician chooses this therapy (Table 5-3). One of the oldest is nitroglycerin or similar medications. These medications can be taken orally, sublingually (under the tongue), or transdermally (by patch or ointment on the skin). They

Table 5-3. Treatments for Stable Coronary Artery Disease

- Medical therapy
  - Nitrates
  - Beta blockers
  - Calcium-Channel blockers
  - Cholesterol reduction therapy
  - Aspirin
- Catheter-Based therapy
  - Balloon angioplasty
  - Rotational atherectomy (rotablator)
  - Directional atherectomy
- Surgical revascularization
  - Coronary artery bypass

reduce or prevent angina (chest pains) by lowering the blood and filling pressures of the heart and by dilating (expanding) the heart arteries and helping balance oxygen supply and demand. These medications can only be used for 12–14 hours per day because the body does not respond to them if they are used continuously. They can cause headaches and light-headedness. There is no evidence that these medications prolong life.

Beta blockers

The beta blockers (propranolol [Inderal]), atenolol [Tenormin], metoprolol [Lopressor], etc.) are another group of medications used to treat angina. These drugs reduce your symptoms by lowering the heart rate and blood pressure and by partially blocking the effects of epinephrine on the heart. In addition to reducing symptoms of CAD, they help prevent irregular heartbeats. For people who have had heart attacks, these drugs dramatically prolong life over the first 3–5 years after the heart attack. Beta blockers may also prolong life in some people with congestive heart failure.

Beta blockers can give some people problems. People with type 1 diabetes who are prone to low blood glucose need to check their blood glucose often because beta blockers can impair the body's response to and warning signs of low blood glucose. People with type 1 and type 2 diabetes may find that beta blockers upset their blood glucose control. The drugs may raise serum triglycerides while lowering HDL (good) cholesterol. They may make peripheral vascular disease worse. People with asthma or other forms of lung disease associated with wheezing may not be able to tolerate these drugs because they can make wheezing worse. Beta blockers may also slow the heart rate too much in patients who already have a low heart rate.

Calcium-channel blockers

The third major class of drugs for angina are the calcium-channel blockers (nifedipine [Procardia], verapamil [Calan], diltiazem [Cardizem], amlodipine [Norvasc], etc.). These drugs treat angina by reducing blood pressure and dilating the coronary arteries. Some of the drugs in this class also reduce heart rate. Dilating the coronary arteries and reducing blood pressure and heart rate balances the oxygen supply and decreases angina. These drugs may allow you to exercise without causing angina. However, use of these medications in people with diabetes is under attack and both short- and long-acting types may have long-lasting consequences for you and should be used with caution.

What else can you do?

It is critical to treat as many risk factors for CAD as possible. Diabetes should be tightly controlled to help prevent damage to organs such as your heart and kidneys.

If your doctor finds cholesterol plaque (buildup), especially in the coronary blood vessels, your cholesterol levels are too high. Cholesterol levels can be controlled in part with careful attention to diet, weight control, and exercise. The use of drugs is often needed, too. The newest class of drugs for lowering cholesterol are called *statins* (lovastatin [Mevacor], pravastatin [Pravachol], simvastatin [Zocor], fluvastatin [Lescol], and atorvastatin [Lipitor]). Large-scale scientific studies have shown that treatment with the statins helps to prevent the development of heart disease and reduces the risk of more cardiac events in those who have already had one.

To further reduce your risk of heart disease, you need to control your blood pressure, lose weight, and stop smoking. There is strong evidence to suggest that long-term treatment with aspirin helps prevent heart attacks. There is also some evidence that eating foods containing antioxidants (vitamins A, C, and E) may be beneficial in preventing or delaying the development of CAD, which is a good reason to add more vegetables and fruits to your meal plan. Try vegetables with deep colors, such as carrots, sweet potatoes, tomatoes, spinach, broccoli, cantaloupe, pumpkin, apricots, and citrus fruits. The main food sources of vitamin E are vegetable oils, green and leafy vegetables, wheat germ (which must be refrigerated because it spoils quickly), whole-grain products, nuts, and seeds.

Will you need angioplasty or bypass surgery?

If you and your physician decide that *cardiac revascularization* (repair or bypass of abnormal coronary arteries) is necessary, several options are available. There are procedures to open the artery mechanically (angioplasty) or to bypass the obstruction in the blood vessel and get the blood flowing again. Studies show that bypass yields better results for people with diabetes.

Angioplasty

A balloon attached to a catheter is inserted into the narrowed artery and inflated to open it. The balloon is inflated many times during the angioplasty to increase the likelihood of the artery staying open. When the balloon is expanded, the cholesterol deposit is reshaped and there is usually a small, controlled tear in the lining of the blood vessel.

Most laboratories have begun to use *stents* with some angioplasties. A stent is a small device, usually made of metal in the shape of a spring or mesh cylinder, that is positioned in the coronary artery at the site of the obstruction. It is compressed until the balloon inflates it to hold the vessel open and prevent the cholesterol deposit from blocking the artery again.

Some blood vessels cannot be dilated with a balloon with or without a stent. These blockages may be opened with a *rotablator*, which has a motorized burr (much like a dentist's drill) located at the tip of the catheter. Some *atherectomy* devices actually remove some of the cholesterol plaque. With both the rotablator and the atherectomy devices, stents are frequently used, too.

Recent data suggests that an angioplasty has adverse affects on people with diabetes. There are serious complications. In some cases, the coronary vessel that has been dilated will re-close abruptly because of clotting at the site of the dilation or tearing of the vessel. Nearly all patients who have angioplasty, with or without stents, receive drugs to prevent clotting.

A stent appears to reduce the likelihood of the vessel closing abruptly. Without stents, as many as one-third of the vessels that are opened may renarrow over 3–9 months. However, even when stents have been used, the blood vessels of people with diabetes are more likely to renarrow after angioplasty.

Bypass surgery

The decision about whether to perform angioplasty or coronary bypass surgery often depends on technical factors, such as the size of the opening in the coronary arteries, whether the obstruction is on a curve or at a branch point, whether there is calcium in the wall of the vessel, and whether the heart pump function is normal. People with diabetes often have diffuse CAD and small openings in the vessels, making angioplasty difficult to do. Success rates are lower in patients with diabetes. Their opened blood vessels are more likely to close up again.

For many diabetic patients, coronary artery bypass surgery is chosen, because it is effective for patients with extensive CAD and those with less serious disease but depressed heart pump function. **Studies have shown that bypass is much more successful than angioplasty in people with diabetes over time.** During bypass surgery, an artery taken from the inside of the chest wall or veins removed from the leg are used to bypass the narrowed portion of the vessel and deliver blood beyond the blockage. This procedure relieves symptoms of angina, may help damaged heart muscle to improve its pumping ability, and, in some patients, may prevent heart attack and prolong life. As with many of these procedures, people with diabetes have lower success rates and earlier return of angina.

The veins used for bypass grafting are usually removed from the lower portion of one or both legs, depending on how many bypasses are necessary. The surgical procedure may require 4–6 hours, or even longer if it is a repeat procedure or if a heart valve must be repaired or replaced at the same time. Complications of bypass surgery include heart attack, bleeding, infection of the breast bone (sternum), or infection of the site from which the veins are taken. Complications are more frequent in people with diabetes, especially postoperative wound infection and difficulties with healing of the breast bone. However, most people with diabetes have coronary artery bypass surgery with excellent results. Typical mortality rates for all patients having bypass surgery in the 1990s are less than 2%.

What is a heart attack?

A heart attack occurs when a coronary artery is clogged or blocked suddenly. Before the heart attack occurs, there may be a gradual blockage of a coronary vessel with cholesterol plaque, as we discussed earlier in this chapter. The difference between stable CAD and a heart attack (myocardial infarction, or MI) is that during the heart attack, one of the cholesterol plaques has cracked, causing a hemorrhage that blocks the vessel, or the vessel can gradually narrow until a tiny clot or clump of platelets can block it and deprive the muscle downstream of the blood necessary for survival. Sometimes, some of the cells that line the coronary artery are sheared off by a rapid blood flow or some other damaging process. The tissue that is exposed promotes vigorous clotting that can block the vessel suddenly. Sometimes blood flows into the exposed cholesterol plaque and shears off a portion of it, forming a flap valve that suddenly blocks the vessel. However the blockage occurs, it prevents blood from reaching some of the heart muscle, causing part of that muscle to die.

What are the symptoms of a heart attack?

Classically, a heart attack presents with a sudden onset of severe, crushing chest pain located under the sternum (breast bone) and spreading to the left armpit, arm, shoulder, neck, and jaw (Table 5-4). If pain is rated on a 1–10 scale, with 1 being very mild and 10 being the worst pain ever experienced, heart attack pain is often 8–10. At the beginning, the pain may be less severe and may come and go over a period of hours, but severe pain is common. The pain can be associated with nausea, vomiting, sweating, palpitations, and shortness of breath.

Sometimes people will have only abdominal discomfort or back pain. And women may have symptoms different from those in men. If a heart attack is suspected, you (or your family) should call an ambulance to take you to the nearest hospital. Speedy transport to the hospital is critical because 50% of all people who die of heart attack do so within the first hour. Many of these early deaths are preventable with prompt medical attention. The earlier treatment is given, the more heart muscle can be saved.

People with diabetes often have different or no symptoms of heart attack. Silent heart attacks are common. If you have several risk factors for heart disease, be alert for any heart attack symptoms, including sudden out-of-control blood glucose levels. Discuss with your doctor whether you need any tests. Heart attack is common in people with diabetes—30–50% more common than in other people of similar age, sex, and risk factors. The risk of having another heart attack is increased for people with diabetes, and the risk is higher for people with type 1 than for those with type 2 diabetes. It is not unusual for people with diabetes to have the symptoms of nausea and

Table 5-4. Symptoms of Heart Attack

- Crushing chest pain
  - Left anterior chest
  - Movement to left shoulder, neck, jaw
  - Bandlike pain/tightness
  - Persistent, more than 15 minutes
- Shortness of breath
- Nausea/vomiting
- Sweating
- Palpitations
  - Fainting
  - Near fainting

shortness of breath but no chest pain because of damage to the sensory nerves of the heart.

How is a heart attack diagnosed?

A heart attack can be diagnosed with an ECG. It can also be detected by blood tests, because with injury to the heart muscle, certain proteins from the damaged heart leak into the blood. Some of these proteins are unique to the heart and provide an extremely accurate diagnosis. The level of these proteins in the blood indicates the magnitude of the heart injury. During hospitalization for heart attack, you may have a cardiac catheterization performed to determine whether angioplasty or coronary artery bypass surgery is appropriate. You may have an echocardiogram and a stress test to evaluate overall heart pump function and to assess your risk for more heart attacks after you are discharged. If you have poor pump function and/or inducible ischemia (imbalance between oxygen supply and demand of the heart), you are at substantially increased risk for another heart attack.

What is the treatment for heart attack?

The first treatment of patients with heart attack is to interrupt the process of the heart attack and get blood flowing to save some of the heart muscle that would otherwise die (Table 5-5). The sooner blood flow is reestablished, the more heart muscle is saved, and the fewer long-term complications there will be. You may be given clot-dissolving medications administered intravenously (through a vein), such as tissue plasminogen activator (TPA) or streptokinase, or you may have an immediate angioplasty.

The decision of whether to use medication or angioplasty is often determined by technical factors, such as the availability of a catheterization laboratory and whether you have conditions that clot-dissolving medications would make worse, such as a recent stroke, bleeding, or surgery (including retinal laser treatment).

If clot-dissolving medications are given within 1 hour of the onset of symptoms, mortality rates can be cut in half. This therapy opens clotted vessels equally well in all patients regardless of whether they have diabetes. Likewise, the complications of thrombolytic therapy, including bleeding and stroke, are the same for all patients. After the clot dissolves, some people have follow-up angiogra-

Table 5-5. Treatment for Heart Attack

Initial
• Thrombolysis (clot dissolver)
• Immediate angioplasty
• Aspirin
• Beta blockers
Long term
• Beta blockers
• Angiotensin-converting enzyme inhibitors
• Cholesterol reduction
• Aspirin
• Risk factor modification
— Smoking cessation
— Hypertension management
— Diabetes management
— Exercise

phy and angioplasty. This is not recommended for people with diabetes, because this approach puts you at three times the risk of complications, including death.

Several follow-up therapies have been studied extensively. The use of beta blockers has been shown to prolong life after heart attack in all patients. Drugs that prevent progressive cardiac enlargement and lower blood pressure (angiotensin-converting enzyme inhibitors, or ACE inhibitors) successfully lower the risk of death over the first 3–5 years after a heart attack for all patients, regardless of diabetes. Long-term therapy routinely includes the use of aspirin, cholesterol reduction, and smoking cessation and should be implemented in all patients.

What is congestive heart failure?

Congestive heart failure (CHF) is a condition in which the heart is unable to pump sufficient blood to meet the needs of the body, particularly kidney function. When this occurs, the body retains water. Symptoms are shortness of breath, decreased ability to exercise, and swelling of the feet and ankles. CHF is a common illness, with 400,000 new diagnoses each year in the U.S. and nearly 3 million people in the U.S. who currently have it. CHF is even more common in the elderly, doubling with each decade over the age of 45 years. It is the leading and most expensive cause of hospitalization in patients over the age of 65 years.

How are diabetes and CHF connected?

If you have diabetes, you have an increased likelihood of developing CHF, because of other cardiovascular problems linked with diabetes, including CAD, heart attack (MI), and hypertension, all of which can cause CHF. However, in the Framingham study, which has followed the heart status of patients over many years, even after all patients with CAD and rheumatic heart disease (heart valve disease) were excluded, the risk of developing CHF was increased four to five times in patients with diabetes. The increased risk was still observed after the effects of age, blood pressure, and cholesterol levels were taken into account.

It appears that diabetes has negative effects on both contraction and relaxation of the heart beyond any difficulties caused by CAD or hypertension. The small vessels of the heart may be affected by diabetes, just as the small vessels in the kidney, the eye, and other organs are affected. Studies of the hearts of diabetic patients who have died have shown a thickening of the walls of the small vessels of the heart and scarring around these vessels as well. Studies of the blood flow of the heart using advanced nuclear medicine imaging techniques have shown that the small vessels of the heart cannot dilate well even in response to powerful drugs. These studies suggest that the small vessels of the heart are abnormal in anatomy and function.

Diabetes affects both the pumping and filling properties of the heart. The heart's inability to pump blood forward makes you feel fatigued even before you exercise. If your heart can't relax, it is difficult for it to fill during the resting phase of a cardiac cycle. This is reflected by high pressures in the heart, which lead to increased blood filling the lungs (backup of fluid). This process makes it difficult for you to breathe, particularly when lying down but also during exercise. The body's attempts to compensate can lead to further fluid accumulation, ankle and leg swelling, and racing and irregular heart rhythms.

How is CHF diagnosed?

The diagnosis of CHF depends on your history of shortness of breath, reduced ability to exercise, and swollen feet and ankles (Table 5-6). The diagnosis is usually confirmed with a chest X ray and a cardiac ultrasound examination (echocardiogram). The echocardiogram allows the cardiologist to distinguish between poor forward heart pump function and increased heart stiffness or poor relaxation—patients often have both. The distinction is important because the treatment for poor forward pump function may be different from the treatment for problems with relaxation.

The most common problem is poor forward pump function. This is usually treated with a combination of medications, including digoxin to increase the force of the heart's contraction, diuretics to help remove excess fluid from the body, and ACE inhibitors (Table 5-7). ACE inhibitors help patients with heart failure by blocking the production of a hormone (angiotensin II) that causes some arteries to constrict. The body constricts these arteries to direct the blood flow to organs that need it most (brain, heart, kidney). Unfortunately, the body's response is excessive and increases the work the heart must perform at a time when it is failing and cannot handle

Table 5-6. Symptoms of Congestive of Heart Failure

- Shortness of breath
  - With exercise
  - When recumbent
- Awakening from sleep
  - For shortness of breath
  - To urinate
- Easy fatiguability
- Swelling of the feet, ankles, and legs
- Palpitations

the extra work. Treatment with ACE inhibitors relaxes some of these arteries, allowing the heart to work more effectively. Treatment of CHF with drugs of this class (enalapril [Vasotec], captopril [Capoten], ramipril [Altace], etc.) reduces symptoms, hospitalizations, and mortality in a wide range of patients. ACE inhibitors must be used cautiously in patients with abnormal kidney function, but they have been shown to preserve kidney function in people with diabetes who have albumin in their urine.

How will treatment of heart problems change in the future?

There are frequent advances in management of heart disease spanning every aspect of cardiovascular disease, diagnosis, and treatment. These improvements apply equally to all patients regardless of whether they have diabetes. New stress testing procedures are being developed to improve the accuracy of the diagnosis of CAD so that fewer patients need cardiac catheterization and coronary angiography. These new advances include new nuclear (radioactive) tracers, nuclear imaging devices, contrast

Table 5-7. Treatment for Congestive Heart Failure

- **Management of underlying cause**
  - — Angina/CAD
  - — Hypertension
  - — Valvular heart disease
- **Digoxin**
- **Diuretics**
- **Angiotensin-converting enzyme inhibitors**
- **Salt restriction**

agents for use with echocardiography, and the use of magnetic resonance imaging (MRI) to assess coronary artery anatomy and heart pump function.

New devices are being introduced almost monthly to improve on angioplasty and stent procedures. In addition, new oral medications are being introduced for the treatment of angina and hypertension. Heart failure management is changing rapidly with the introduction of beta-blocker therapy and other new hormone-blocking agents that seem promising. The pace of change in the diagnosis and management of heart disease is rapid and has already improved short- and long-term outcomes.

This chapter was written by Edward M. Geltman, MD.

6

Cholesterol and Other Blood Fats

Case study

Mr. and Mrs. JS, a couple in their early 50s, have made an appointment with their physician to discuss their risks of heart attack and blood vessel disease. Their concern was triggered by Mr. JS's brother having a heart attack. Also, his father had died of a heart attack.

Introduction

Coronary heart disease (CHD) is a disease of the blood vessels supplying the heart. It is the primary cause of death in the U.S. Every minute, an American suffers a heart attack, and about 500,000 people die of CHD each year.

Even though a heart attack is a catastrophic event, the process leading up to a heart attack (called *atherosclerosis*) develops over several years. *Athero* refers to a deposit of gruellike soft, pasty material, and *sclerosis* means to harden. Atherosclerosis is a slow process of fatty substances such as cholesterol building up and coating the inside of the arteries. This process occurs at a faster rate in individuals with high blood cholesterol, diabetes, or high blood pressure or those who smoke. As a result of this accelerated process, blood vessels become narrowed to the point where they are no longer able to supply sufficient blood to organs such as the heart or brain. (See chapter 5 on heart disease and chapter 7 on stroke.)

A rupture of the fatty plaque releases substances that cause an instantaneous clot in the blood vessel. This is the most common cause of heart attacks (about 70%). The remaining 30% of heart attacks are caused by progressive narrowing of the arteries. Narrowed arteries cause a decrease in the blood flow and lack of oxygen to the cells of the heart. The limited blood flow causes pain, which we call angina.

What is cholesterol?

Cholesterol and other blood fats belong to a family of molecules called lipids. Blood fats include substances called triglycerides, and they actually form the fatty tissue in the human body. Fats are unique in that they do not mix well with water, and they have to be packaged with water-soluble proteins to form lipoproteins to be transported in the blood. Cholesterol and fats are essential parts of all cell membranes and have several important functions:

- to form insulation around nerves
- to make bile, which is necessary for absorbing fat and fat-soluble vitamins
- to serve as an important source of energy

Where do you find cholesterol and fat?

The cholesterol that the body needs is made mostly in the liver. The rest comes from what you eat. An average American eats a diet that is 45% carbohydrates, 15% protein, and about 40% fat. Egg yolks and organ meats are particularly rich in cholesterol.

How is the energy from fats different from the energy from carbohydrates and protein?

Triglycerides are made up of a molecule of glycerol attached to three fatty acid molecules. These are very efficient sources of energy. Compared by weight, fat can generate twice as much energy as either protein or carbohydrate. By cutting the amount of fat you eat, you save calories but still get the same amount of energy that you would from protein or starches, and you will be eating less of certain kinds of fatty acids that contain the building blocks necessary for making cholesterol in the body. All this makes your blood fat levels healthier.

What are saturated fats?

These are fats that harden at room temperature and are found in animal products such as beef, veal, lamb, pork, butter, cream, and whole milk. They are also found in shortening, coconut oil, and palm oil. If you eat too much of these substances, they are stored as fat and also increase the production of cholesterol in your body.

What are polyunsaturated and monounsaturated fats?

These are oils that are liquid at room temperature. The oils that contain polyunsaturated fats include sunflower, soybean, cottonseed, and corn. Monounsaturated fats are derived from canola and olive oils and actually cause a reduction in cholesterol. However, even these so-called good oils cause weight gain when you eat too much of them.

What are the different types of cholesterol?

As noted above, cholesterol is packaged into lipoproteins to be transported in the blood. Based on the way the cholesterol and protein are packed together and the amount of cholesterol that the lipoproteins contain, they can be classified into different kinds—high-density lipoprotein (HDL), low-density lipoprotein (LDL), and triglycerides.

What are high-density lipoproteins, or HDL?

These fats are made in the liver and intestine and contain very little cholesterol. They serve to collect excess cholesterol from the blood and blood vessels and transport it back to the liver, where it is broken down. HDL is sometimes called the "good" cholesterol. The higher your HDL level, the better. The American Diabetes Association (ADA) recommends that you aim for an HDL level greater than 35 mg/dl.

What are low-density lipoproteins, or LDL?

These lipoproteins contain a very high concentration of cholesterol and carry the cholesterol from the liver throughout the body. This form of cholesterol is also the culprit responsible for the buildup in the walls of the arteries that leads to atherosclerosis. Some people call it the "bad" cholesterol. The higher the concentration of this form of cholesterol in the blood, the greater the chance of getting CHD. A desirable level of LDL depends on whether you already have CHD and whether you have other risk factors that would predispose you to developing CHD. LDL levels should be below 130 mg/dl. If you already have CHD, your LDL level should be less than 100 mg/dl.

What are triglycerides?

These are a form of fat that is carried in the blood but is mostly stored in fat tissue. The ADA goal is a level less than 200 mg/dl. Higher levels are usually found in people with diabetes, and they can play a relatively minor role in the development of CHD. Some people believe that high triglycerides are an important risk factor for CHD in women. Very high levels (greater than 1,000 mg/dl) are dangerous and can cause pancreatitis (inflammation of the pancreas).

How can I tell whether I have high cholesterol?

Unfortunately, in the early stages, it is a silent disease very much like high blood pressure. You often find out about high cholesterol when you start having chest pain or, worse still, after a heart attack. Rarely, with some hereditary forms of high cholesterol, people develop "bumps" on the skin and tendons at the elbow and ankle, and a physician might notice these during a physical exam. You should have your blood tested to measure your cholesterol at regular intervals. It is better not to wait until CHD is advanced enough to cause chest pain.

When should I be tested for high cholesterol?

Cholesterol testing is recommended for all individuals over the age of 20 and every 5 years thereafter if they have desirable cholesterol levels (see below). The first test to be done is a measurement of total cholesterol (and HDL cholesterol if possible). This test does not require you to fast. If
- your total cholesterol is more than 240 mg/dl
- your cholesterol is between 200 and 230 and you have two or more of the risk factors listed below
- you already have CHD

then you need to have an additional test to determine the blood fat levels of LDL and triglycerides. This test is called a lipoprotein profile and requires you to fast beforehand. Fasting means you may not have anything to eat or drink except for water, black coffee, or tea without milk, cream, or sugar for 9–12 hours before the test, which should be done first thing in the morning.

What factors make cholesterol high or low?

The factors that can affect your cholesterol levels are heredity, age, sex, diet, weight, exercise level, alcohol intake, cigarette smoking, hypertension, and diabetes.

Heredity

Your genes can influence your cholesterol levels. If your parents have high cholesterol levels, you probably will, too. One specific form of inherited condition called *familial hypercholesterolemia* affects 1 in 500 people and can lead to early CHD.

Age and sex

Cholesterol levels increase with age. Women are protected by their female hormones (estrogens) until menopause, but women with diabetes lose this protection. Men older than 45, women older than 55, or post-menopausal women at any age should consider themselves at higher risk for CHD, especially if they have diabetes. (See chapter 5 on heart disease.)

Diet

Foods high in cholesterol and saturated fat raise your LDL levels. In fact, it is believed that eating foods high in these substances is the main reason for the high incidence of CHD in the U.S. compared with the rest of the world.

Weight and exercise

Excess weight, which is usually in the form of fat, increases LDL levels. Weight reduction not only decreases your LDL and triglyceride levels, it increases your HDL levels. The same benefits can be gotten from regular physical activity. You can make a difference!

Alcohol

Small quantities of alcohol can raise your HDL, the good cholesterol, as you may have learned from advocates of the "Mediterranean diet," which recommends a daily glass of wine for a healthy heart. Drinking too much alcohol can increase your triglyceride levels and cause liver damage. Alcohol should not be your main defense against CHD.

In addition, the following act as risk factors for CHD on their own:

- cigarette smoking
- hypertension
- diabetes

What are the benefits of lowering cholesterol?

Several research studies have been conducted to see whether lowering your cholesterol leads to a reduction in the number of heart attacks. Most of these were done in patients who already had CHD, in whom lowering cholesterol clearly prevents second heart attacks and lowers the risk of dying from one. Separate analyses of just the patients with diabetes in these studies show that the benefits of lowering cholesterol are even more dramatic than in the patients without diabetes. A few studies also showed that the same holds true even for people without previous CHD. One major study was conducted in about 4,000 patients followed for 5 years. They found that by lowering LDL with a group of drugs called *statins*, there was a 42% reduction in the number of deaths from heart attacks and a 37% reduction in the chance of having a heart attack.

Based on the results of this study, for every 1,000 patients who are treated for 5 years and have their cholesterol levels lowered to the same extent,

- 40 people would be saved who would otherwise die from CHD
- 70 of the 210 expected heart attacks would be prevented

When this is extrapolated to the approximately 3.5 million Americans with CHD and high cholesterol levels similar to those in the study, cholesterol lowering would prevent about 140,000 deaths, 270,000 heart attacks, and 585,900 hospitalizations for CHD.

What does your cholesterol mean to you

Because your diabetes puts you at greater risk for CHD, you want your cholesterol levels to be as close to normal as possible. Your total cholesterol level should be less

Table 6-1. Desirable Cholesterol Levels

Type	Cholesterol Level (mg/dl)
Total cholesterol	
• Desirable	<200
• Borderline	200–239
• High	>240
HDL	
• Desirable	>35
• Low	<35
LDL	
• If you already have CHD or have diabetes	<100
• If you have >2 risk factors	<130

> means greater than
< means less than

than 200 mg/dl. Your HDL should be 35 mg/dl or more, the higher the better on this one. The desirable level of LDL depends on whether you have CHD or any other risk factors. In every instance, the best way to achieve desirable blood fat levels is with a balanced meal plan and daily exercise (see Table 6-1).

What should you do once you know you have high cholesterol?

Based on Table 6-1, you and your doctor should set your cholesterol (especially LDL) goals. You can affect your cholesterol levels with changes in your meal plan, level of exercise, and weight and by taking cholesterol-lowering drugs. Of course, it is most desirable to control your cholesterol levels without the use of drugs, if possible.

What changes can you make in your diet?

Changes in diet help reduce cholesterol and are one of the most effective means of reducing your weight. The best—and perhaps only—way to get a meal plan that fits you and your lifestyle is to see a registered dietitian (RD) and work together.

1. **If you do not have CHD, you have fewer than two risk factors, and your LDL level is more than 160 mg/dl,** follow a Step I diet prescribed by an RD. This is not just a list of foods to avoid. In this diet, saturated fats provide no more than 8–10% of the calories, and cholesterol content should be less than 300 mg/day. If LDL does not decrease to less than 160 mg/dl in 3 months, you should proceed to a Step II diet. This diet has less than 7% of total calories from saturated fat, and the cholesterol content is less than 200 mg/day. Typically, if you follow a Step II diet, you can expect about a 10–15% reduction in LDL levels. If there is no

improvement even after 6 months on this diet, you may need to begin drug therapy.

2. **If you do not have CHD but have more than two risk factors,** then your LDL goal is less than 130 mg/dl. You should follow the same steps as above.

3. **If you already have CHD,** then your LDL goal should be less than 100 mg/dl. You should begin a Step II diet immediately, and if your goals are not met within 6–12 weeks, you should start drug therapy.

4. **If you have diabetes,** your LDL should be less than 100 mg/dl.

How can exercise affect your cholesterol level?

Physical activity helps in reducing weight, increases HDL levels, and improves other risk factors such as diabetes and hypertension. This could be aerobic exercise such as walking, biking, jogging, or swimming for at least 30 minutes, four times a week. An exercise program should be tailored to you, especially if you have recently suffered a heart attack. Check with your physician before you start an exercise program, and get the assistance of an exercise physiologist or other qualified professional. Exercise can worsen eye and kidney disease, raise blood pressure, damage feet, cause a heart attack, or raise or lower blood glucose levels. Be sure you understand how the exercise you choose will affect any complications you may have.

How does weight control affect your cholesterol level?

Weight loss of 5–10 pounds can lower your cholesterol level another 5–10%. For a weight-loss program to be successful in the long term, it needs to be reasonable. If you aim at reducing your meal plan by about 500 calories per day, you will have a healthy weight loss of 1/2 to 1 pound a week. An RD can help you design or adjust your meal plan. You should not go below about 1,200 calories a day. If you want to keep eating the same amount but still lose weight, try exercise. Remember that increasing your daily activity is the way to burn calories. Muscle tissue, which you build up as you get in better shape, burns calories even when it is at rest.

When will your physician begin drug treatment?

If your LDL level remains above your goal, despite your best efforts at the above measures for at least 6 months, then drug treatment should be considered. You must continue to follow a good diet and exercise program even if you begin drug therapy. Several drugs are now available for this purpose. As is the case with most medications, these drugs have side effects, and you should be closely followed by your physician. Some of the drug classes that are commonly used are statins, bile acid resins, nicotinic acid, fibric acid derivatives, and hormones.

Statins

These drugs inhibit the enzyme that controls the rate at which cholesterol is produced in the body by the liver. They also improve the ability of the liver to remove LDL cholesterol from the blood. They apparently stabilize the plaque that lines the arteries, thereby helping to prevent ruptures that lead to clots and heart attacks.

Currently, there are five statin drugs in the U.S. market: lovastatin (Mevacor), pravastatin (Pravachol), simvastatin (Zocor), fluvastatin (Lescol), and atorvastatin Lipitor). All of these agents are equally effective in bringing LDL levels down by about 20–60%. These drugs are given as a single dose at bedtime. Effects are seen in about 4–6 weeks, which is why your lipid profile (blood test) should be repeated at about this time. Serious side effects are rare. Mild gastrointestinal symptoms, including abdominal cramps, gas, and constipation, usually go away after the first few weeks. Periodic laboratory testing should be done to watch for abnormalities in liver function. Rarely, some people may develop soreness and weakness of muscles. If this develops, you must stop your medication immediately and see your doctor.

Bile acid resins

These agents bind cholesterol in the intestines, and this combination is then eliminated in the stool. The bile acid resins lower LDL cholesterol by about 10–20%. Cholestyramine and colestipol are the two main drugs available in this class. They can be combined with statins for an additive effect on cholesterol reduction. Their greatest advantage is their safety profile, because they are not absorbed into your system. Bothersome side effects include constipation, bloating, and gas. These side effects can be avoided by taking the drug with meals and with large quantities of water. They can also cause your triglyceride levels to increase, so this will need to be watched. In addition to binding to cholesterol, bile acid resins interfere with the absorption of other medications taken at the same time. The other medications should be taken at least 1 hour before or 4–6 hours after the resin.

Nicotinic acid

Despite the favorable features of this medication, nicotinic acid is often avoided in patients with diabetes because it increases blood glucose levels. It is actually a B vitamin and has several beneficial effects, such as causing a 10–20% reduction in LDL cholesterol and a 20–50% reduction in triglyceride levels. It also raises HDL levels by about 15–30%. This drug is inexpensive and available without prescription. However, because of potential side effects, it should not be used without a doctor's supervision. The immediate-release form is preferred, and the dose should be started low and raised slowly. A common side effect is flushing, which can be reduced by taking aspirin first. Discuss this with your doctor.

Fibric acid derivatives

Gemfibrozil (Lopid) is the fibric acid derivative available in the U.S. and is mainly effective in lowering triglyceride levels by about 20–50%. These agents are often used in people with diabetes who have elevated triglyceride levels.

Hormones

The risk of CHD is greater for postmenopausal women. Estrogen replacement raises HDL levels, lowers LDL levels, eliminates fat from the bloodstream, increases blood flow throughout the body, and helps keep blood vessels flexible. So it is often offered to postmenopausal women who do not have breast cancer or a history of blood clots in the legs. Estrogen does have side effects. High doses are associated with increased chance of breast or uterine cancer. If a woman has her uterus, she needs to also take progesterone to oppose the effects of the estrogen. If a woman does not have a uterus, she can take estrogen without progesterone (Estradiol, Estraderm, or Premarin). Estrogen can cause the blood to clot more easily, putting you at increased risk for a stroke. With low doses, 0.625 mg or less, of Premarin this is not a problem. The chance for stroke is higher in women with high blood pressure and those who smoke.

Hormone therapy works for some women and doesn't work for others. It can cause extremely high triglyceride levels in some people. Women on hormonal therapy should be watched for this, because it can cancel out the other benefits of these drugs for your heart. Progesterone, used in combination with estrogen, can cause you to feel anxious, depressed, or edgy. You may take estrogen in three forms: an oral tablet, a vaginal cream, or a patch worn on the skin. The vaginal cream does not affect cholesterol levels. Estraderm, the patch, does not increase HDL cholesterol but does decrease LDL levels. Discuss whether hormone therapy would be a good choice for you with your health care provider.

Aruna Venkatesh, MD, and Laurinda Poirier, RN, MPH, CDE, contributed to this chapter.

7

Stroke

Introduction

Diabetes increases your risk of having an ischemic stroke. An ischemic stroke is caused by a lack of blood supply to an area of the brain—without evidence of bleeding, which can also cause a stroke—because of blockage of a blood vessel either in or leading to the brain. Your risk of brain hemorrhage is not higher because you have diabetes, so this chapter deals specifically with ischemic stroke. Diabetes does increase your risk of ischemic stroke by approximately two to three times. This increased risk of stroke is present whether you have type 1 or type 2 diabetes. Diabetes increases the risk of stroke regardless of other risk factors, such as high blood pressure.

People with diabetes also tend to have more severe disabilities after stroke, a higher frequency of recurrent stroke, and a higher risk of death after stroke than the general population. However, your risk of stroke can be reduced by knowing the warning signs and by identifying risk factors other than diabetes that you can modify. There are medications and a surgical procedure called *carotid endarterectomy* that can be used to reduce the risk of stroke in appropriate situations.

What are the signs and symptoms of stroke?

A stroke is an episode where there is a change in the blood supply to a particular part of the brain. The brain is an organ that requires a lot of oxygen to maintain normal functioning. The brain receives and requires a constant blood supply circulated from the heart to the brain arteries. When there is an interruption in the blood supply to an area of the brain, dysfunction of that part of the brain occurs. There are certain warning signs and symptoms that indicate that a temporary (transient ischemic attack, or TIA) or permanent (stroke) lack of blood supply is occurring in the brain. This is best illustrated by the following case:

A 65-year-old woman with a history of type 2 diabetes, hypertension, and hyperlipidemia (elevated blood fats or lipids) went to her physician for an episode of "drooping" of the right side of her face, weakness in her right arm, and difficulty with her speech that lasted 15 minutes and resolved earlier that day. She reported a blood glucose level of 180 mg/dl after the episode. Her physician told her that he was glad she came for evaluation so quickly. He listened to her carotid arteries (in her neck) and her heart and performed a neurological examination. He heard a left carotid bruit (a soft, whooshing sound) over the artery in her neck. He recommended further testing, including a carotid artery ultrasound; a complete blood evaluation that included testing her blood glucose, cholesterol, and triglycerides; and a brain computed tomography (CT) scan. He started her on aspirin, which can prevent clotting.

In approximately 20% of people who go on to have a stroke, there is a preceding TIA that is a clear warning sign of a possible impending stroke. A TIA usually lasts 5–15 minutes and then resolves. It differs from a stroke in one regard, and that is the short, reversible duration of the symptoms. A TIA is an important sign to pay attention to because if a person is treated after it occurs, the risk of a subsequent stroke is reduced.

There are typical warning signs of a TIA or stroke (Table 7-1). One of these signs is sudden weakness or numbness of the face, arm, or leg, usually on one side of the body. Rarely, there may be involvement of both sides of the body at the same time. The weakness may be described as heaviness or clumsiness of the arm and/or leg. There may be weakness of one side of the face, often described by the person as "drooping." There may be sudden dimness or loss of vision, particularly in one eye. This may be described as a "fog," "haze," or "scum" over the eye. The loss of vision may progress from the top to the bottom of the vision in one eye. Speech may be slurred (referred to as *dysarthria*). Individuals with this symptom have trouble pronouncing words clearly or articulating. Other people have trouble understanding words that are spoken, trouble expressing themselves, or difficulty in both areas. There may be difficulty reading or

Table 7-1. Warning Signs of a Stroke

- Sudden weakness or numbness of the face, arm, or leg on one side of the body
- Sudden dimness or loss of vision, particularly in one eye
- Loss of speech or trouble talking or understanding speech
- Unexplained dizziness, unsteadiness, or sudden falls, especially with the presence of any of the above symptoms
- Sudden, severe headaches with no apparent cause

writing. The broad term for problems in these areas is *aphasia* (literally meaning "without speech"). Sudden onset of spinning dizziness (vertigo), unsteadiness of walking, or rarely, a sudden fall can be warning symptoms of an impending stroke. Typically, these symptoms do not occur in isolation and may be seen in association with visual dimming or loss in both eyes, double vision, or slurred speech. Finally, a sudden, severe headache with no other apparent cause can be a stroke warning symptom. Headaches accompany ischemic stroke approximately 20% of the time.

What are the causes of stroke in a person with diabetes?

In the U.S., approximately 500,000 people experience a stroke each year. The rate of stroke in people with diabetes is approximately 60 strokes per 1,000 people with diabetes, while the rate is approximately 30 strokes per 1,000 people without diabetes. The risk is present in both men and women with diabetes but is greater in women. In men with diabetes, there is a 2.5-fold higher incidence of ischemic stroke, and in women with diabetes, there is a 3.6-fold higher incidence. Although stroke can affect any age-group, the greatest risk of stroke in people with diabetes is to those in their 50s and 60s.

Stroke can be divided into ischemic stroke and hemorrhagic stroke. An ischemic stroke is the most common type of stroke, accounting for approximately 80% of all strokes. This type occurs when there is blockage of blood flow to the brain due to blockage of an artery or arteries (Figure 7-1). There can be many reasons for an artery being blocked, the most common of which is *atherosclerosis* (fat or lipid deposits called *plaques* on the artery walls). Atherosclerosis of the arteries occurs more commonly, advances more rapidly, and is present at a younger age in

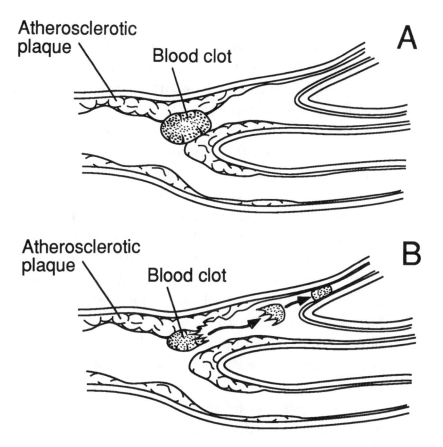

Figure 7-1A. In an area of atherosclerotic narrowing of a blood vessel, a blood clot can form and block off the blood vessel, often leading to a stroke. **B.** A blood clot can originate in the area of an atherosclerotic plaque or it can travel from the heart to the blood vessel. A piece of the clot can break off and lodge in a smaller artery, causing a stroke.

people with diabetes compared to those without diabetes. Atherosclerosis is just as common in women and men with diabetes. Important risk factors, in addition to diabetes, that can contribute to the development of atherosclerosis include hypertension, elevated blood fats or lipids, and smoking.

Atherosclerosis can affect the large arteries traveling to the brain (macrovascular disease) or the small arteries within the brain (microvascular disease). In people with diabetes, there is more extensive atherosclerosis of both the large arteries in the neck (extracranial arteries) and the arteries that travel into the brain (intracranial arteries). In addition, there are important racial and sex differences in the distribution of large-artery disease. Caucasian men tend to have more disease of the extracranial large arteries. African-American men, women, and some Asian groups tend to have more intracranial disease. There is a type of stroke called a *lacune* that is a small (less than 1 cm) infarction deep in the brain or brain stem that is typically due to disease of the small brain arteries. Hypertension is the most common risk factor for a lacunar infarction. Some studies have shown that diabetes may be associated with lacunar infarcts. Diabetes has been associated with changes to the small cerebral blood vessels. However, the degree to which this causes the development or affects the outcome of stroke is not clear.

Another cause of ischemic stroke, called *cardioembolism,* is often due to the development of a clot in one of the chambers of the heart that subsequently breaks loose and lodges in an artery of the brain. This type of event causes 15–20% of all strokes. Other conditions that contribute to this type of stroke are numerous. The most common are atrial fibrillation (an irregular rhythm of the heart due to rapid and ineffective beating of the atria of the heart) and history of heart disease, such as a prior heart attack, history of rheumatic fever with valvular abnormalities, or congestive heart failure. In a person with diabetes, a heart attack, which at times may go unrecognized by the individual, or a heart that is not contracting properly because of disease of the heart muscle (cardiomyopathy) can lead to this type of stroke.

Another cause of stroke in people with diabetes is having something wrong with the blood, referred to as a *hematological* abnormality. There may be abnormalities in the way the blood clots caused by changes in clotting factors, platelet adhesiveness (stickiness) and aggregation (clumping), or the way red blood cells change their shape as they travel through the blood vessels. Sickle-cell disease is another such clotting disorder. The end result is a *hypercoagulable* state, which means that the red blood cells can clot more easily than normal. Hematological abnormalities are seen especially in people with diabetic kidney disease (nephropathy) (see chapter 9).

Does diabetes affect what happens after you have a stroke?

People with diabetes have a higher rate of death, a worse neurological outcome, and more severe disability after stroke than those without diabetes. The death rate in people with diabetes 1 year after stroke is 50%, compared to 25% in those without diabetes. One reason for poor long-term outcome after a first stroke in people with diabetes is the high frequency of recurrent stroke. An elevated blood glucose on admission to the hospital is one way to predict that a person's condition will deteriorate after stroke. Despite conflicting results from studies, most experimental studies in animals indicate that hyperglycemia (high blood glucose levels) increases the extent of brain damage due to ischemic stroke. One study has shown that stroke patients with admission glucose levels greater than 150 mg/dl developed more brain swelling after stroke as measured by brain CT scan than did people with glucose levels less than 100 mg/dl. However, elevated blood glucose may be a reflection of how severe the stroke has been rather than being a contributor to the outcome after stroke. It is not clear whether control of elevated glucose levels can affect the outcome after stroke.

How does your physician diagnose stroke and determine the cause?

Stroke is a diagnosis that is made on the basis of the sudden onset of a neurological impairment that may include numbness, weakness, visual loss, speech changes, coordination or balance difficulties, vertigo (spinning dizziness), or impaired memory.

A 50-year-old man with a 30-year history of type 1 diabetes was diagnosed with a stroke by his physician because of the development of weakness of the left side of his face and left arm. His physician explained to him that certain tests needed to be done to determine the cause of his stroke—a scan to image the brain, cardiac testing, a carotid ultrasound, and a blood evaluation.

Testing that may be done to detect a stroke includes a brain CT (or CAT) scan or magnetic resonance imaging (MRI) of the brain. A CT scan of the brain quickly creates several images of the brain within approximately 10 minutes. Images that are produced help the doctor determine whether the stroke is caused by bleeding (hemorrhage) or blockage (ischemia). MRI of the brain uses a large magnetic field and radio waves to produce a three-dimensional image of the brain without the use of radiation. This test can accurately identify small areas of stroke in places the CT may not show, such as the brain stem, cerebellum, and deep in the brain hemispheres. An MRI takes longer than a CT to perform. It is not as well tolerated by some people after stroke either because of their illness or because of claustrophobia in the MRI chamber.

A CT is the usual test that is done immediately after a stroke to determine whether there is bleeding, which would change the way the doctor manages you after stroke. A carotid artery duplex scan is an ultrasound of the neck arteries that can determine whether there is stenosis (narrowing) or total blockage of the carotid arteries in the neck. Cardiac testing may be done, including an electrocardiogram (ECG), to check for an abnormal cardiac rhythm, or an echocardiogram, which is an ultrasound of the heart done to check for any clots in the chambers of the heart or other abnormalities that could be the source of a stroke. Specialized testing of the blood is indicated to rule out a metabolic or hematologic abnormality responsible for stroke. In people with diabetes, blood tests for serum glucose, serum cholesterol, and triglycerides are particularly important. Low blood glucose (hypoglycemia) can sometimes mimic a stroke or cause a seizure with paralysis. This usually resolves quickly after the low blood glucose is treated, but in some cases, the symptoms may last for several days. The purpose of the basic tests is to try to determine a cause of the stroke, which directs the physician toward the appropriate treatment to prevent a recurrent stroke.

What happens after you have a stroke?

After an acute stroke, you are admitted to the hospital, preferably to a dedicated acute stroke unit under the care of a neurologist. It may be necessary to consult an endocrinologist, internal medicine physician, or family physician for appropriate management of diabetes or for control of hypertension. Depending on the type of neurological impairments that are present after stroke, other health care professionals may be consulted, including a dietitian, speech pathologist, physical therapist, occupational therapist, and recreational therapist. After a stroke, the person may need intensive rehabilitation under the care of a physician specializing in physical medicine. It is also important to check for and quickly treat any depression that may be present.

How can you prevent an initial or recurrent stroke?

Anyone who wants to prevent a stroke needs to consider modifying the treatable risk factors, initiating medical therapy, and/or having surgery.

What are the risk factors for stroke?

There are a number of conditions called risk factors that increase the risk of stroke. Minimizing your risk of stroke is possible by treating or eliminating the risk factors you can change. However, there are some risk factors that you cannot change, called unmodifiable risk factors. Knowing about these risk factors is important. If diabetes is combined with other risk factors, the risk of stroke can rise significantly.

What are the risk factors that you can't change?

Age

Age is the greatest risk factor for stroke in anyone. The incidence of stroke increases with age. Almost 75% of strokes occur after age 65. In fact, the risk more than doubles with each decade after age 65.

Sex

Stroke is more common in men than in women until the eighth decade of life. While men are at a greater risk for stroke than women at most ages, stroke continues to be a major killer of women. Women are catching up with men as far as stroke risk because of factors such as smoking, especially smoking while using birth control pills. Women with diabetes are at higher risk than men with diabetes.

Race

African Americans are approximately 60% more likely than Caucasians to have a stroke. It is likely that both genetic and environmental factors play a role. The presence of obesity in African Americans, Hispanics, and American Indians causes their risk of developing diabetes to increase significantly, which may be one factor that leads to an increased stroke risk. Part of the high stroke risk in African American women has been related to a higher prevalence of hypertension and diabetes in that group.

Family history

Heredity can play a role in the risk of developing stroke. This is particularly true if hypertension, diabetes, or abnormal blood lipids are particularly prevalent in a family.

What are the risk factors that you can change?

Hypertension

Elevated blood pressure is the major risk factor for stroke. Unfortunately, more than half of the people with hypertension do not even know they have it. High blood pressure is defined as a blood pressure measurement with the systolic (upper number) greater than 140 mmHg or the diastolic (lower number) greater than 90 mmHg on several different readings. People with diabetes have a 40% higher incidence of hypertension. If hypertension is combined with other risk factors, such as obesity, high blood lipids, smoking, or diabetes, the risk of stroke is greatly increased. The successful treatment of hypertension has contributed to the decline of the number in strokes and deaths from strokes in recent years.

Elevated blood lipids

The link between elevated blood lipids (fats) and stroke is not as clear as the association with heart disease. It is clear that elevation of blood lipids accelerates the development of atherosclerosis, which can lead to stroke.

Cardiac disease

There are many different cardiac diseases that can increase the risk of stroke. Some of the more common causes are heart attack, congestive heart failure, rheumatic heart disease, artificial heart valves, and atrial fibrillation or other heart-rhythm disturbances.

Tobacco

Cigarette smoking increases the risk of stroke dramatically. Men who smoke have a 40% greater chance of having a stroke than do nonsmokers. Women who smoke have a 60% greater chance of having a stroke compared with nonsmokers. If a woman smokes and uses birth control pills, her risk of stroke is increased 22 times. Smoking or exposure to secondhand tobacco smoke increases the chances of developing atherosclerosis.

Alcohol

Heavy or binge drinking is strongly associated with stroke. Alcohol increases blood pressure levels, which increases the risk of stroke.

Drugs

Drugs, including cocaine, LSD, and amphetamines, can increase blood pressure and cause stroke. Substances in the drugs can also have toxic effects on the blood vessels that can lead to stroke. Oral contraceptives have been shown to increase your chances of having a blood clot that could lead to a stroke.

Diabetes

Studies have shown that the risk of stroke in people with diabetes is approximately two to three times greater than in people without diabetes.

Does good blood glucose control help you prevent a stroke?

While there are studies addressing the question of whether good control of blood glucose can reduce the risk of stroke, no definitive answer to this question is available yet. Therefore, it is uncertain whether diabetes is a modifiable or unmodifiable risk factor. The presence of diabetic complications such as coronary artery disease, disease of the blood vessels in the legs (peripheral vascular disease), diabetic kidney disease (nephropathy), and disease of the blood vessels in the eyes (retinopathy) has been linked in some studies to a greater stroke risk. Being aware of the risk factors that you have that are treatable or modifiable is the first step toward minimizing your risk of stroke.

What are the medical treatments for stroke?

There are three categories of treatments available for prevention of stroke or recurrent stroke. These include medical therapy with platelet antiaggregants, including aspirin or ticlopidine (Ticlid); anticoagulants, such as warfarin (Coumadin); or surgical intervention with a procedure called carotid endarterectomy.

Platelet antiaggregants

Platelet antiaggregants work by preventing the blood platelets from sticking together and forming clots. The most commonly used agents in this category are aspirin and ticlopidine (Ticlid). Aspirin has been used for several decades to reduce the risk of stroke. Studies have shown that aspirin reduces the risk of nonfatal stroke by 30%, the risk of nonfatal heart attack by 30%, and the risk of death by 15% compared with groups taking a placebo. Aspirin has the advantages of being inexpensive, generally safe, and well tolerated by most individuals. The most common side effects are gastrointestinal irritation or bleeding. The dosage recommended by physicians in the U.S. varies between 81 and 1,300 mg/day. The appropriate dose for you should be recommended by your physician. If you are allergic to aspirin or cannot tolerate it, you should inform your doctor so that an alternative medication may be prescribed.

Ticlopidine (Ticlid) is another platelet antiaggregant. While ticlopidine differs from aspirin in the way it affects the platelets, the end result is prevention of blood clotting by keeping the platelets from sticking together. It is a more potent inhibitor of platelets than aspirin. In people with diabetes, ticlopidine has been shown to significantly inhibit platelets from sticking together. It has the added benefit of slowing the progression of background retinopathy (nonproliferative diabetic retinopathy). In general, physicians usually recommend ticlopidine for patients who have continued TIAs or a stroke despite aspirin therapy or in patients who do not tolerate aspirin or are allergic to it. Ticlopidine is more expensive than aspirin.

Some of the side effects seen with ticlopidine are diarrhea, skin rash, and a reduction in the number of infection-fighting white blood cells in the body (*neutropenia*). Neutropenia develops in nearly 1% of patients and is reversible if it is detected promptly. For this reason, when this medication is prescribed, blood tests to detect this potentially fatal side effect are done every 2 weeks for the first 3 months of therapy.

Anticoagulants

Anticoagulants, or blood thinners, such as heparin or warfarin (Coumadin), are another form of medical therapy that are given to prevent stroke or recurrent stroke. In general, anticoagulants are used in patients who have strokes caused by cardiac clots that break loose and lodge in the brain arteries (*cardioembolism*).

In other instances, anticoagulants are given when patients fail to respond to platelet antiaggregants. Heparin is a medication that is given intravenously or by injection for a short period after a stroke to prevent the blood from clotting. It is usually administered in the hospital setting immediately after a stroke. Although it is not of proven value after a stroke, it is sometimes given to prevent further clot formation or to prevent clotting in an area of tight narrowing of a blood vessel.

Warfarin (Coumadin) is another anticoagulant that works by preventing the blood from clotting by inhibiting the production of some of the clotting factors in the liver. Warfarin is of proven value in prevention of stroke in people with atrial fibrillation. It may also be used after some types of myocardial infarction (MI, heart attack) to prevent stroke. It is not uncommon for patients to be given both heparin and warfarin for several days after an acute stroke, followed by the use of warfarin alone once the desired degree of blood thinning is reached. The main potential side effect of these agents is bleeding, either into the brain or at other sites in the body. The degree of thinning of the blood needs to be carefully and frequently monitored with blood testing. Check with your physician about the foods and medications that can affect the warfarin dose. The effectiveness of warfarin compared to aspirin in prevention of recurrent stroke caused by hardening of the extracranial and intracranial arteries is being closely studied.

What is the surgical treatment for stroke?

Carotid endarterectomy is a surgical procedure used to treat atherosclerotic narrowing of the carotid arteries in the neck. In this procedure, the carotid artery is opened, and the layer of plaque (buildup) in the artery is removed. Recent studies have provided some guidelines for performing carotid endarterectomy in people after a stroke. In patients with symptoms, either TIA or mild-to-moderate stroke, surgery is highly beneficial if there is 70–99% narrowing (stenosis) of the carotid artery on the same side as the symptoms. The results for patients with symptomatic 30–69% narrowing of the carotid artery are not available yet. It has been determined that carotid endarterectomy is not beneficial for symptomatic patients with less than 30% carotid artery narrowing or in people with complete (100%) blockage of the carotid artery.

This surgical procedure is not indicated in patients who are at a high risk for surgical complications, such as those with poor heart or lung function. Only people who are good candidates for surgery are considered for the procedure. People with diabetes are at increased risk for early postoperative cerebral complications. In addition, people with diabetes undergoing surgery who have severe retinopathy, neuropathy, nephropathy, congestive heart failure, disease of the heart valves, or disease of the peripheral blood vessels are at an increased risk for complications, including stroke.

This procedure is also recommended in some individuals with 60% or greater narrowing of the carotid artery and no symptoms of stroke (asymptomatic carotid artery stenosis) to reduce the subsequent risk of stroke.

What are the recent advances and future treatment for stroke?

In the last few years, there have been some exciting advances in the area of stroke treatment. Some guidelines for the use of carotid endarterectomy have been determined. There are many new drugs that are being studied for stroke prevention and management of stroke after it has occurred.

One promising new therapy is tissue plasminogen activator (TPA). TPA is a thrombolytic agent (literally, a substance that dissolves a clot) that is used intravenously within 3 hours after the onset of stroke symptoms. The availability of this drug has placed an increased emphasis on the need for emergency management of stroke. TPA is only for people with ischemic stroke (no brain hemorrhage). There are strict and specific guidelines for the use of TPA after stroke.

There are experimental studies involving a procedure called angioplasty. In this procedure, a small flattened balloon is inserted into a blood vessel. In the region of narrowing or blockage, the balloon is expanded to try to open the passage. Studies are evaluating whether this will

Table 7-2. How to Reduce Your Risk of Stroke

- Know the warning signs of stroke and obtain emergency treatment if they occur.

- Pay attention to the modifiable risk factors, including hypertension, elevated blood lipids, and cardiac disease. Avoid tobacco, alcohol, and illicit drugs.

- See your physician regularly. Be compliant with treatments for high blood pressure and heart disease and with any treatment given to you by your physician for prevention of stroke.

be a good treatment for patients with narrowing of cerebral blood vessels.

In summary, the risk of stroke is increased if you have diabetes. People with diabetes are two to three times more likely to have an ischemic stroke, and they are more likely to die from the stroke. However, treating the other risk factors and using medical or surgical treatments can reduce your risk of stroke.

This chapter was written by Jose Biller, MD, FACP, and Betsy B. Love, MD.

8

Hypertension

Introduction

Hypertension means high blood pressure. If you have hypertension and diabetes together, you are at higher risk for cardiovascular and kidney disease.

Mr. LJ is a 43-year-old African-American senior executive who was sent by his company for a health check-up. A few months ago, he was told that he had elevated blood pressure, but because he was feeling fine, it was not treated. He works very hard in a stressful environment. His typical day starts around 8:00 A.M. after a traditional American breakfast of eggs, bacon, and buttered toast. He is so busy that he hardly has time for lunch and usually eats a bag of potato chips or a king-sized candy bar. He finishes work around 7:00 P.M. and spends the evenings with his family having a large dinner and watching TV. He gets little exercise, traveling by car and using the elevator at the office. Mr. LJ smokes a pack of cigarettes daily. He enjoys drinking alcohol but does not use any other recreational drugs. Fortunately, he has not had any major medical illnesses in the past. Both his mother and father have hypertension and diabetes, and his father has had a major heart attack from which he almost died. Mr. LJ is 5 feet 8 inches tall and weighs 250 pounds.

DR. JR: Your blood pressure reading today is high. You told me that a few months ago another doctor recorded high readings. Before I say that you have hypertension, I would like to confirm at least two more readings, a week apart.

MR. LJ: I have heard that some people have high blood pressure only in the doctor's office. Is that what is happening to me?

DR. JR: That is called "white coat hypertension," where people have high blood pressure readings in the doctor's office but normal readings at home. We need to measure your blood pressure at home several times. I will lend you a blood pressure monitor and stethoscope and teach you and your wife how to use them. Then I will see you in a week. With your medical and family history and your lifestyle, you are at risk for high blood pressure, diabetes, elevated blood cholesterol and lipids, and cardiovascular disease, which are all serious diseases. You will have the laboratory screening tests for these. The results should be available the next time we meet.

One week later

DR. JR: Welcome back, Mr. LJ. I have the results of your home blood pressure readings and lab tests. You do indeed have hypertension. Your blood chemistries indicate that you may also have diabetes and elevated blood cholesterol.

MR. LJ: Is this a common problem?

DR. JR: Yes. There are approximately 16 million people with diabetes in the U.S. and 30–40 million people with hypertension. Nearly 3 million people have both diseases. You are one of them. So you see, this is a common problem. The causes are both hereditary and environmental. As people age, they are more likely to develop both hypertension and type 2 diabetes. When we consider race, African Americans are almost twice as likely to have diabetes and hypertension, and Mexican Americans are three times more likely to have them than the general population.

MR. LJ: What causes hypertension in people with diabetes?

DR. JR: Hypertension in people with diabetes is usually *essential hypertension* (no cause is found). This is particularly true of type 2 diabetes. We do know that between 35 and 75% of all diabetic complications result from hypertension. It is well worth your time to check what causes yours. Hardening of the arteries, or *atherosclerosis* (the process of cholesterol building up on the blood vessel wall), may narrow the arteries supplying the kidneys. This causes high blood pressure, called *renovascular hypertension*, which is potentially correctable. In a recent autopsy study, 73% of patients with narrowed renal arteries had hypertension and 53% had diabetes.

MR. LJ: When do you say a person has hypertension?

DR. JR: Hypertension is not diagnosed on a single measurement but on high readings on at least two occasions, a week apart. The National High Blood Pressure Education Program report on high blood pressure in diabetes suggests an average of 90 mmHg (or greater) diastolic or a systolic blood pressure of 140 mmHg (or greater) for a diagnosis of hypertension.

MR. LJ: Once you have established that a patient with diabetes has hypertension, what next?

DR. JR: I ask the patient the following questions:

1. Tell me what medications, prescribed and over the counter, you are taking. I want to see whether any of these might contribute to high blood pressure or diabetes. Over-the-counter medications that may raise blood pressure include certain pain medications like ibuprofen, cold and sinus remedies, appetite suppressants, and some drugs used in treating depression.

2. Do you have abnormal blood cholesterol or lipid levels? What were your previous test results?

3. Do you smoke cigarettes?

4. Do you have heart disease, stroke, kidney disease, or eye disease? Have you ever suffered a heart attack? Have you ever had a cardiac (heart) stress test? If so, what were the results?

5. Do other family members have heart disease, hypertension, diabetes, or kidney disease?

6. Do you get cramps in the calves of your legs when you walk short distances?

7. Describe your dietary habits. Do you add salt to prepared foods? Do you consume a lot of canned foods and processed meats? These usually contain large amounts of salt, which raises blood pressure in some salt-sensitive people. Describe your use of alcohol.

8. Do you exercise? If so, what kind? How often?

9. Have you gained or lost weight recently? How much weight and why do you think you lost it?

10. Do you have numbness or tingling in your hands or feet?

11. Have you had any episodes of impotence? Have you had frequent urinary tract infections? Are you unable to empty your bladder when urinating?

12. Do you become dizzy when you stand up?
   For already established patients, I ask:
13. How long have you had diabetes and hypertension?
14. What treatments have you received in the past? How did you respond to them? List any side effects you had.
15. Have you been told you have leakage of albumin or protein in the urine?
16. When was your last eye exam? What was the result?

MR. LJ: You said you would perform a physical exam. What are you looking for?

DR. JR: Apart from recording your height and weight, I would like to measure your blood pressure when you are standing, sitting, and lying down on your back two or more separate times (at different visits). This is because there is a greater variability in blood pressure measurements in people with diabetes. It will also give me an opportunity to determine whether you are one of those patients whose blood pressure drops when they stand up. The condition is called *orthostatic hypotension* and is especially difficult to treat. Also, some medications used to treat hypertension may cause orthostatic hypotension as a side effect, particularly in people who have diabetes.

I will then examine your neck for distended veins, which may signify heart failure. I will listen with my stethoscope on your neck (on both sides of your windpipe) for a bruit—the sound of blood flowing through narrowed neck arteries that supply blood to the brain. This gives a clue about the presence of vascular (blood vessel) disease. Then I will use a hand-held ophthalmoscope to examine the retinas of your eyes, and I will check those blood vessels for evidence of disease resulting from diabetes and/or hypertension.

I will carefully examine your heart for enlargement and other effects of hypertension, such as hypertrophy (thickening of the wall due to excess work) and failure (inability to cope with excess demand). I will listen to your lungs to check for the congestion that accompanies heart failure. I will listen to your abdomen for bruits (as in the neck). These sounds come from narrowed renal arteries (arteries that supply the kidneys). I will check for masses in the flank areas (to detect enlarged kidneys, which may suggest polycystic [containing many cysts] kidneys) and distended urinary bladder. Diabetes can affect the nerves to the bladder (autonomic nervous system disease). (See chapters 9 and 12.)

I will carefully examine your feet to detect diminished or absent pulses, which suggest peripheral vascular disease (small blood vessel disease; chapter 10), and swelling of the feet and legs (*edema*, caused by fluid building up in the tissues), which may suggest you have heart or kidney failure or side effects from some medications. I will check your nervous system for nerve damage. Peripheral nerve disease with numbness and tingling in the feet is confirmed by loss of feeling. A sensitive method of testing for this is to use a vibrating tuning fork at the base of the big toe. I'll also use a monofilament to test your ability to feel a light touch. We'll do these tests every time I see you.

The results of my examination may show a correctable cause for hypertension. These results can include flank masses, suggesting enlarged polycystic kidney disease; bruits heard especially in the diastolic (the relaxation period of the heart) phase; or bruits heard in the abdomen, suggesting high blood pressure in the blood vessels in the kidneys. I do not find any organ damage. Therefore, I assume that you have not had high blood pressure for long

MR. LJ: Could you explain what tests you performed?

DR. JR: Before I begin a treatment and at the time of diagnosis, I request a series of blood tests that include serum creatinine (a marker of kidney function), TSH (a thyroid test), electrolyte levels that may point to hypertension caused by excess production of certain hormones, a CBC (complete blood count) to check for anemia, and a glycated hemoglobin (HbA_{1c}) to measure your blood sugar levels over the past 2–3 months. A fasting serum lipid profile to detect abnormalities in your cholesterol levels (cholesterol, HDL, LDL, and triglycerides) is also important for patients with diabetes and hypertension.

A complete urinalysis will detect any proteinuria (protein leaking into the urine) or other problems. This will include a 24-hour collection of urine to check for small amounts of protein (called *albumin*) that might not show up in the single urine sample.

We will repeat some of these tests 6–12 weeks after treatment is begun to see the effects of medication, especially on blood lipids. These are tests that you should have at least yearly, but the type of tests and how often you have them should be based on the damage to your organs and how you respond to the selected treatments. You may need other specialized tests or consultations.

MR. LJ: Will I need to see any specialists?

DR. JR: Having determined that you do not have organ damage, I'll refer you to an ophthalmologist for now. I recommend this for adult patients when they are diagnosed with diabetes (see chapter 4).

I am also going to have you see a registered dietitian (RD). You will need a carefully planned diet because you have diabetes, hypertension, and elevated blood lipids (loosely termed *cholesterol*). The RD will help you develop a meal plan with foods you choose for meals and snacks that will supply the total calories you need and help you lose weight.

I also want you to see Ms. DF, a registered nurse clinician specially educated and certified in diabetes education (a certified diabetes educator, or CDE). She will teach you how to check your blood glucose and blood pressure at home and help you deal with specific situations. You can call her when you have questions.

MR. LJ: What symptoms do patients with hypertension usually have? Why didn't I have any symptoms?

DR. JR: Most patients with hypertension have no symptoms. You are a classic example. By the time symptoms appear, organ damage has often set in. The symptoms are from the damaged organs themselves. Physicians have to be on the lookout and screen for hypertension periodically. This is usually done during annual physical exams, employment physicals, or ordinary visits to health providers for some other cause such as an acute illness. Certainly, if a patient has a family history of heart disease, kidney disease, diabetes, or hypertension, routine screening is necessary.

MR. LJ: How do I go about managing my problems?

DR. JR: There are several phases to managing your health problems. You'll need to make some lifestyle changes. As I told you earlier, you have diabetes, hypertension, and elevated blood lipids. What you eat is a key factor in your management. You are overweight, and losing weight plays a major role in controlling all three problems. You'll be encouraged to know that you will start seeing significant benefits even after losing only a few pounds. You do not have to reach an ideal body weight to see results.

Exercise is as important as food. The type of exercise should be aerobic—walking, jogging, bicycling, swimming, or rowing. You should not do high-intensity exercises, such as weight lifting done with a bearing-down motion or holding your breath, which increase the strain on the heart and elevate blood pressure. (You probably can lift light weights and build strength with more repetitions, but get instruction from a qualified teacher.) You don't want more harm than good to come from your exercise. It is important to get medical advice before you begin an exercise program. I'd like you to see Dr. MM, a cardiologist and exercise physiologist, who may perform an exercise stress test to check how your heart performs during exercise. Remember, you should start slowly, progress gradually, and report any symptoms such as chest pain and shortness of breath immediately. Don't just rely on the exercise test results.

MR. LJ: What do you mean by lifestyle changes?

DR. JR: Diet and exercise are the most important ways that we define our lifestyle—the way we choose to live. Changing these two significantly affects your health. Other powerful lifestyle changes are stopping cigarette smoking completely, using alcohol in moderation, and reducing stress. If you make all of these changes, you'll take control of all three medical conditions and prevent complications.

MR. LJ: I have read somewhere about nonpharmacological treatments. What are those?

DR. JR: The name means treatment without the use of drugs. This is actually a different way to describe those lifestyle changes, such as avoiding tobacco and eating less fat. I usually try nonpharmacological treatment alone for a period of 3 months if the initial blood pressure readings are not very high (generally lower than 160/95 mmHg).

However, if you have organ damage, risk factors like elevated blood lipids, diabetes, cigarette smoking, obesity, sedentary lifestyle, or family history of premature cardiovascular disease, I may prescribe drug therapy at the time of diagnosis. You fall into this category. However, I strongly recommend that you make the lifestyle changes, too. If you succeed with nonpharmacological measures, you'll require smaller amounts of medication to control your blood pressure. You may also reduce side effects from the drugs and find it's easier to take them. Lifestyle changes will help increase your chances for successful step-down therapy (reducing dosage and/or number of drugs) after your blood pressure has been well controlled for more than 1 year on at least four consecutive office visits.

MR. LJ: Since you have made it clear that I will need drug therapy, I'm curious about how you choose the right drug combination for me. Are specific drugs indicated for specific patient groups? Please explain.

DR. JR: The Joint National Committee for Hypertension has extensively reviewed several treatment approaches to hypertension. The combination of hypertension and diabetes carries a greater risk of target organ damage than does either disease alone. That's why there are special qualifications for when to use hypertension drug therapy for people with diabetes.

1. Patients with diabetes and hypertension who have blood pressure of 140/90 mmHg or higher are candidates for drug therapy to reduce blood pressure to 130/85 mmHg or less.

2. The presence of complicating kidney disease limits drug choices because of the effects of each drug on kidney function and diabetic nephropathy.

3. Some drugs can upset blood glucose and blood lipid levels.

4. Orthostatic hypotension is common in people with diabetes and needs to be remembered when choosing which drugs to use.

   In clinical trials, only beta blockers and diuretics have been shown to decrease death from cardiovascular disease. I tend to use beta blockers only under special circumstances, for example, in patients with diabetes and hypertension who have angina or after a heart attack, where it can prevent sudden death. Diuretics are better known as water pills. There are several classes of these drugs depending on how and where in the kidneys they act. I won't go into the complex actions of these drugs. Generally, there is no reason to use diuretics except thiazides for the treatment of hypertension. Thiazide diuretics in low doses (25 mg/day or less) have acceptable side effects and generally work for people with diabetes. Because diuretics can cause potassium loss, you would need frequent tests of blood potassium and may need a potassium supplement.

Another recommended class of drugs for patients with diabetes and hypertension is the *converting enzyme inhibitors*. These agents are based on the principle that there is an enzyme chiefly in the lung (but also in other tissues) called angiotensin-converting enzyme, or simply ACE. ACE converts angiotensin I to angiotensin II, which has strong effects on blood vessels, constricting them and elevating blood pressure. By successfully blocking (inhibiting) the action of this enzyme, these drugs reduce blood pressure. That's why they are called ACE inhibitors. They also have several other beneficial effects. Most important, they reduce proteinuria and slow the progression of diabetic kidney disease. They do not affect blood glucose control and do not raise blood lipids, but these drugs are not without side effects. ACE inhibitors in rare instances can worsen kidney function in patients with narrowing of both renal arteries. Therefore, we would need to monitor serum creatinine and potassium. We must take care when combining therapy with diuretics because the drop in blood pressure can be deep. Cough is a common side effect of ACE inhibitors.

Another class of drugs to treat hypertension in people with diabetes is the calcium-channel blockers, also known as calcium antagonists. These drugs generally do not raise blood glucose or lipid levels. However, they should be used with caution because they may bring on orthostatic hypotension. Some members of this group of drugs (especially nifedipine) can worsen proteinuria and increase the heart rate. **Generally, they should not be used.**

A class of drugs called alpha blockers has also been recommended. Like beta receptors, there are alpha receptors in the blood vessels. Blocking alpha receptors makes the blood vessels relax, thereby decreasing their resistance and lowering blood pressure. These drugs do not affect blood glucose levels. They may also have a beneficial effect on blood lipids. Caution is needed when beginning these agents, because the very first dose can cause a sharp drop in blood pressure. I usually warn patients of this and start them on the lowest dose. I ask the patient to take the medication at bedtime and advise caution when rising. These drugs may also help patients with enlargement of the prostate and difficult urination by relaxing the urethra. This is an example of the two-for-one concept—a drug is selected not only for its effect on blood pressure but also for its effect on coexisting diseases or symptoms.

A new class of agents, the *angiotensin II receptor blockers,* is now available. These drugs block the effect of angiotensin II and are very effective in lowering blood pressure. They significantly reduce proteinuria, improve blood lipid levels, and don't cause side effects like coughs. There is no dosage adjustment necessary for patients with kidney disease, and needing to take them only once a day improves the likelihood of patients remembering to take them.

MR. LJ: All this talk about drugs makes me wonder how much lifestyle changes can reduce blood pressure.

DR. JR: In a study called TOMHS (Trial of Mild Hypertension Study), lifestyle changes alone reduced average blood pressure from 141/91 to 130/83 mmHg for 234 participants after 1 year.

MR. LJ: Would you recommend lifestyle changes for normal people?

DR. JR: Yes. It would make everyone healthier and happier. I would recommend lifestyle changes to everyone, especially those with blood pressure in the high-normal range (systolic 130–139 and diastolic 85–89 mmHg) to keep them from developing high blood pressure in the future.

MR. LJ: You mentioned earlier that the presence of diabetes and hypertension worsens the target organ damage more than either disease does alone. Could you explain this with specific examples of the target organs?

DR. JR: I'm glad you asked. Let's take cardiovascular disease. The risk to your heart and blood vessels is doubled when you have diabetes and hypertension. This includes coronary heart disease (which produces heart attacks), heart failure, and peripheral vascular disease, causing poor circulation in arms and legs, which can end in amputation. The risk of strokes is increased by two to four times in people with diabetes. Hypertension increases the risk by six times. Thus, the risk of stroke is substantial when you have both diseases.

Eyes are another target. Eye disease (retinopathy) can be affected by diabetes and hypertension. Patients with both diseases are definitely at higher risk for optic nerve damage and glaucoma. Systolic blood pressure (the top number) is a predictor of the frequency of it happening, and diastolic blood pressure (the bottom number) predicts the progression of retinopathy. Retinopathy is twice as likely to occur when the average systolic blood pressure is 145 versus 125 mmHg. Diabetic retinopathy is the most frequent cause of new cases of blindness in American adults aged 20–74 years. Good control of hypertension can go a long way in preserving eyesight.

Remember how the kidneys can be damaged, a disease called diabetic nephropathy. Hypertension speeds up the progression of this complication. Remember that control of hypertension along with good blood glucose control can prevent the progression of nephropathy. So, you see that controlling hypertension is a key factor in preventing some of the dreaded complications of diabetes.

MR. LJ: Some of my friends who take medicines for blood pressure have problems with their sex life. I am skeptical of taking medications because I feel it may destroy my harmonious family life.

DR. JR: I know you're concerned about the side effects of the drugs, but the diseases themselves can cause sexual problems in both men and women. Certainly, hypertension, neuropathy, vascular disease, and psychological problems can cause impotence, impaired ejaculation, or decreased libido in men (see chapter 17). In women, these complications can result in decreased vaginal lubrication, decreased libido, and difficulty in achieving an orgasm (see chapter 18). Lowering your blood pressure can help prevent these complications.

Certainly, your concern is valid. The drugs can have this side effect, but it should not stop you from taking them for now. Keep an open mind and if this problem does occur in the future, we can adjust your medication to minimize the problem.

MR. LJ: That is very reassuring. Now that I am ready to take on treatment for my conditions, what should I do to be sure that my treatments are successful? Why treatment programs fail and what can be done to make them successful?

DR. JR: Maintaining a long-term effective treatment regimen is not possible without continued commitment by you, your family, and me. Aside from your primary physician—me—other health care practitioners, such as nurses, pharmacists, podiatrists, dietitians, and optometrists, can play vital roles in education and support of you and your family.

I would encourage you to master the skills you need for self-care and follow the treatment plan we are going to develop together. I'll try to make the instructions simple and clear. I'll also write them down so that you can refer to them later.

MR. LJ: Why does a program fail?

DR. JR: The major reason is that patients don't make lifestyle changes or take their drugs. Sometimes this is because of the cost of the drug, unclear instructions, instructions not being written down, not enough patient education, or the physician trying to dictate to the patients instead of treating them as partners in decision making.

One helpful strategy is to have the patient sign a written contract with realistic short-term goals. The doctor and patient can review them periodically, taking care not to be judgmental if the program isn't working. Patience and perseverance are the rules for success.

By the same token, a successful patient-education program should be tailored to the patient and be culturally sensitive. The diabetes educator must pay attention to the ethnic, religious, and regional issues of the patients. Adults need hands-on, active learning. And the family should be involved at every stage. They can help record the results of blood glucose and blood pressure monitoring in a simple-to-use log book. The log book should be reviewed periodically with the provider to make treatment decisions. Providers should keep patients aware of available community resources and programs at workplaces and health care institutions.

MR. LJ: Speaking of home monitoring. What kind of blood pressure instrument do you recommend for use at home? How do I interpret the numbers?

DR. JR: The "gold standard" for blood pressure measurement is the mercury sphygmomanometer, but it is more difficult to learn to use. There are new electronic models with increasing degrees of sophistication. You want a monitor that is consistent, accurate, easy to use, and affordable. Your machine should be checked against the one in my office periodically to make sure your home monitoring results are accurate. Whatever instrument you choose to use, make sure you choose an appropriate cuff size, place the arm at the level of the heart, and are well rested before taking measurements. Remember that blood pressure readings vary at different times of the day. In addition, physical activity, stress, caffeine, tobacco, and alcohol can influence readings. Be honest when you write down the results, because you cannot fool the target organs! It is better to stay away from electronic finger models because there are more factors that can interfere and give false readings.

MR. LJ: Are there any separate guidelines for managing patients with diabetes and hypertension among special groups?

DR. JR: I would consider children, pregnant women, and elderly people as special groups. I'll tell you about the elderly patient with diabetes and hypertension. The other two groups are dealt with by specialists. I had mentioned earlier that both diabetes and hypertension increase with age. The elderly patient benefits as much as, if not more than, his younger counterpart from treatment of hypertension. This is true even of the very old (over 85 years) and for elevation of either diastolic or systolic blood pressure.

Elderly patients sometimes have difficulty in metabolizing drugs (because of alterations in blood flow to the liver and decreased kidney function), can't afford drugs, or fail to take their drugs because of decreased memory and dementia. It is wise to start with the lowest drug dose and cautiously and slowly increase it. Drugs have longer duration of action in the elderly than in other groups. Orthostatic hypotension can be a problem, but wearing elastic stockings may help.

MR. LJ: I've heard that some patients have elevated systolic blood pressure alone. Do you recommend treating them?

DR. JR: When such patients (systolic blood pressure higher than 160 mmHg but diastolic blood pressure lower than 90 mmHg) are treated, they can benefit in cardiovascular health. I recommend a small dose of a thiazide diuretic at first. These patients are usually elderly and need to be seen frequently. When beginning treatment, they should be watched for orthostatic hypotension, or low blood pressure, on standing up. If a second drug is needed, I recommend an ACE inhibitor or a calcium antagonist. If the elderly patient also has heart failure, the ACE inhibitor will treat both conditions.

MR. LJ: Could you help me better understand the mechanisms underlying these two diseases?

DR. JR: The likelihood of developing both type 2 diabetes and hypertension increases with age, especially in the African-American population. There is a change in body composition that occurs with aging—a significant loss of muscle and an increase in total body fat. The skeletal muscle is mostly responsible for metabolizing carbohydrates, which may explain why diabetes is strikingly high in the elderly. A particular kind of obesity called *android, central,* or *abdominal obesity* (as opposed to gynoid, or female-like, obesity, where the fat is in the hips) is tightly linked to a number of diseases such as diabetes, hypertension, and coronary artery disease. If your waist and hips are about the same size, you're in this group.

Certain minority groups have specific risk factors. African Americans are more sensitive to salt. Genetic factors count, but social and economic factors play significant roles. Factors include diet, exercise, obesity, and insulin resistance. People in lower socioeconomic classes, particularly women, are much more likely to develop obesity, diabetes, and high blood pressure.

MR. LJ: What promise does the future hold for a patient with hypertension and diabetes?

DR. JR: There are several very promising drugs being studied that lower blood pressure and improve diabetes control. The most promising belongs to the class called thiazolidinediones. The FDA has already approved troglitazone (Rezulin), a drug in this class. These drugs increase insulin sensitivity without stimulating the body to produce more insulin. Indeed, these compounds given over a 12-week period decreased insulin resistance, improved blood glucose levels, and lowered blood pressure in obese people who did not have diabetes. This observation throws further light on and strengthens the theory that obesity, hypertension, insulin resistance, and abnormal blood lipids are interconnected and reflect a common abnormality in the cells that handle metabolism. (People who take Rezulin need to have their liver enzymes checked regularly.)

We need to look for medications that reduce not only blood pressure but also cardiovascular risk and slow the development of diabetic kidney disease. The ACE inhibitors and calcium antagonists have shown some promise in this area. More long-term studies are needed for these drugs. Hopefully, we will learn to manage diabetes and hypertension better to reduce human suffering and lighten the financial burden that these two diseases place on us.

This chapter was written by Venkatraman Rajkumar, MD, and James R. Sowers, MD.

9

Nephropathy

Case study

A 37-year-old woman who has had type 1 diabetes since age 7 noticed ankle swelling and increasing girth over a 6-month period. Over the years, her blood sugar control had only been fair. She had hypertension, and microalbuminuria (small amounts of albumin, a protein, in her urine) had been showing up in her lab tests for the last 2 years. She recently needed laser therapy for proliferative diabetic retinopathy. Her current lab tests showed large amounts of albumin in her urine. Her serum creatinine was 2.1 mg/dl (normal is less than 1.2 mg/dl). When kidneys start to fail, the blood creatinine begins to rise. Her physician diagnosed nephrotic syndrome, a condition of protein loss and water retention. He prescribed an angiotensin-converting enzyme (ACE) inhibitor, a medicine that lowers blood pressure and helps to improve kidney function, and sent her to see a registered dietitian for help in cutting back on the amount of protein and salt that she eats.

Case study

After 11 years of type 2 diabetes, a 54-year-old, African-American man with high blood pressure complained of being unable to concentrate and of constantly feeling cold. Weakness, nausea, a 12-pound weight loss, and itchy skin were also complaints. On physical examination, the patient was found to have advanced renal disease with a serum creatinine of 11.6 mg/dl (normal is less than 1.2 mg/dl). He recently needed laser surgery for diabetic retinopathy, and this added weight to the diagnosis of advanced diabetic nephropathy. The patient, his wife, and his clergyman met to consider whether peritoneal dialysis, hemodialysis, or a kidney transplant was the best option for him. Three brothers and two sisters all offered to donate a kidney.

Introduction

Today diabetes is the leading cause of kidney (renal) failure worldwide. The good news is that the more successful you are at managing your diabetes, the longer and healthier your life should be. The bad news is that a longer life span gives some people with diabetes time to develop the "late" complications of diabetes, including kidney failure. That may be why diabetes now accounts for 40% of all new cases of kidney failure. African Americans, Hispanics, and American Indians (especially the Pima tribe) are three to five times more likely to have both diabetes and kidney complications. Of people with type 1 diabetes, 30–50% are likely to develop diabetic nephropathy after having diabetes for 40 years. In people with type 2 diabetes, diabetic nephropathy is a bit of a mystery. Damage to their kidneys has become a sign that they are at risk for a stroke or heart attack. In groups of people who are very susceptible to type 2 diabetes, such as the Pimas, the rates of nephropathy are about the same as for people with type 1 diabetes.

For all people with diabetes, this is a serious complication to have to consider. However, ongoing research and improvements in diabetes management have resulted in better early treatment programs, which may prevent or slow the disease, and have improved the quality of life of all people afflicted with serious kidney disease.

What do your kidneys do?

The two kidneys are located in the back of the abdomen on either side of the spine. Each is about the size of an Idaho potato weighing about 1/2 pound, and each processes about one-quarter of the blood pumped by the heart. One kidney can do the work for two, which is why people born with only one kidney or who lose a kidney by trauma, disease, or as a transplant donor have a normal life expectancy. Blood flow through the kidney amounts to about one quart every minute. The kidneys' job is to remove nitrogen-rich end products of protein digestion and water and to maintain a balance of sodium and potassium. Like other vital organ systems, renal function has a large reserve capacity.

Each kidney is made up of between 600,000 and nearly 2 million subunits called *nephrons*. Specialists in internal medicine who work primarily with diseases of the kidney are called *nephrologists*. Individual nephrons begin with a complex of tiny blood vessel loops called a *glomerulus*, through which blood from the heart is filtered. The blood is delivered by an *arteriole*—a small artery. Blood, minus what was filtered, leaves through another arteriole to return through veins to the heart. The filtrate enters a long path in the nephron called a *tubule*, where it is changed into urine and discharged into the bladder via the *ureters*—tubes connecting the kidneys to the bladder.

Disease of the kidney (renal disease) is called *nephropathy*, and people with diabetes have *diabetic nephropathy*. However, not all kidney disease in those who have diabetes is related to diabetes. For example, you may inherit a kidney disorder, have a tumor or enlargement of the prostate gland that obstructs urine flow and puts backup pressure on the kidney, or have an infectious disease that affects your kidneys. Certain drugs can also affect kidney function. That is why it is sometimes difficult to determine whether kidney disease is diabetes related or caused by something else.

Who is at risk for developing diabetic nephropathy?

The longer you have diabetes, the more at risk you are for developing diabetic neuropathy. But after 40 years of diabetes, only 30–50% of people with type 1 diabetes develop kidney disease. People whose blood glucose control is not good are more at risk for developing the disease. Some people have a genetic tendency to develop the disease, especially if a near relative has it. People with high blood pressure are more likely to develop nephropathy—and nephropathy makes high blood pressure even worse. Other risk factors include high cholesterol levels, urinary tract infections (UTIs), and smoking.

What are the symptoms of kidney disease?

Unfortunately, kidney disease doesn't have any symptoms until it is pretty far along. That is why laboratory tests need to be done at regular intervals to tell you and your physician how your kidneys are doing before serious symptoms show up.

What are the stages of diabetic kidney disease?

The stages of diabetic kidney disease are hyperfiltration, microalbuminuria, nephrotic syndrome, renal insufficiency, and end-stage renal disease.

What is hyperfiltration?

The first stage of diabetic kidney disease has no symptoms and is called *hyperfiltration*. Early in the course of diabetes, in as many as 70% of those with type 1 diabetes and about 33% of those with type 2 diabetes, an above-normal amount of blood passes through the filtering glomeruli in their kidneys. Kidney size increases early in the development of diabetic kidney disease. Careful regulation of blood glucose levels can, however, reduce kidney size to normal. A kidney function test called *clearance* may show that you are experiencing hyperfiltration, but that does not mean that your kidneys will get worse. Less than 50% of people who have diabetes and hyperfiltration go on to the later stages of nephropathy.

What is microalbuminuria?

Microalbuminuria is the condition of small amounts of a protein called albumin showing up in your urine. Healthy people have less than 25 mg of albumin in their urine each day. Microalbuminuria (30–300 mg/day) occurs in 4–15% of adults with diabetes, typically in those who have had the disease for at least 5 years. Hyperfiltration may not be present with microalbuminuria. It is important to detect microalbuminuria early because people with type 1 diabetes who have microalbuminuria are more likely to progress to the later stages of kidney disease. People with type 2 diabetes who have it are more likely to have a heart attack or stroke. If you have microalbuminuria, you may prevent or slow the development of more serious conditions for many years by bringing your blood pressure down to normal and by achieving good blood glucose control. A specific laboratory test must be done to find microalbuminuria, because the usual urine dipsticks or clinic tests for protein are not sensitive enough. The first morning specimen of urine is the most reliable. If this test is positive, a 24-hour urine specimen should be checked for total albumin content. The result can be compared with the same test taken after treatment is begun, to see whether there has been improvement. Repeat tests need to be taken because the level of albumin in urine naturally varies from day to day for different reasons. It may also be influenced by exercise.

Although microalbuminuria has no signs or symptoms, we know that there are changes in the small blood vessels of the kidneys that are unique to diabetes and that blood pressure increases in the filters in the kidneys. Microalbuminuria signals the need for treatment with ACE inhibitors. ACE inhibitors lower the blood pressure within the glomerulus so that less protein, or albumin, is leaking from the blood into the urine, and they slow the deterioration of kidney function.

What is nephrotic syndrome?

If the injury to the blood filters in the kidneys gets worse, albumin loss in the urine rises to 3,500 mg/day or more and can be measured by a dipstick test. This stage is called dipstick-positive *proteinuria*, or clinical nephropathy. The changes that take place in the kidneys are called the *nephrotic syndrome.*

Because you're losing so much albumin in your urine, the level of albumin in the blood decreases to less than the normal range of about 3.9–4.6 g/dl. This diminishes the ability of the blood to hold plasma water inside the arteries and capillaries. Water then accumulates in the tissues as *edema* and in the chest (*pleural effusion*), around the heart (*pericardial effusion*), and in the abdomen (*ascites*). These are the areas where you may notice symptoms if the disease has progressed this far. Albumin synthesis in the liver is increased to compensate for the low plasma level. This causes the liver to produce more cholesterol and fats (*hyperlipidemia*), which can cause other health problems. In the nephrotic syndrome, fluid is retained in the body, and water weight may reach 50 pounds. Carrying this much extra water causes fatigue and shortness of breath due to fluid in the chest. People with nephrotic syndrome often note that their shoes don't fit and dresses and pants will not button because of the water weight, and even routine activities are difficult and tiring to complete.

What is renal insufficiency?

This stage is called advanced clinical nephropathy or kidney failure. At this stage, the damaged kidney is no longer able to filter toxins from the blood or prevent protein from leaking into the urine. Among the protein wastes proposed as toxins are urea, creatinine, uric acid, phenols, and guanidines. Physicians monitor the condition of the kidneys by blood tests measuring either the nitrogen in urea (blood urea nitrogen, or BUN) or the serum creatinine. More precise estimates of remaining kidney function can be obtained by a clearance test using urine and blood together to measure either creatinine or a radioisotope (radioactive chemical) excreted by the kidney. This test often requires a timed urine collection.

Patients have few symptoms until renal function declines to less than 30% and the serum creatinine and BUN levels are higher than normal. When serum creatinine rises above 2.0, the patient should see a nephrologist. Listlessness, loss of appetite, feeling cold, being unable to concentrate, nausea, and itching are common complaints as kidney failure becomes more severe. Anemia is common. Once renal function declines to less than about 15%, symptoms of kidney failure such as skin bruising, intermittent vomiting, weight loss, somnolence during the day and insomnia at night, restless legs, and lethargy may convert a formerly active individual to a chronic invalid. At this stage, less insulin is needed because less insulin is eliminated by the kidneys.

What is end-stage renal disease (ESRD)?

After months to years of renal insufficiency, renal function decreases to the point where life is no longer possible without major therapeutic intervention. Untreated ESRD may induce major swelling of the bowel and fluid collection into the sac surrounding the heart, thereby limiting its ability to pump blood. Muscle cramps and even death may occur when blood potassium rises because potassium cannot be excreted in the urine. High blood potassium levels affect heart function. Patients may also have convulsions. *Uremia*—Greek for "urine in the blood"—is the term applied to ESRD in its last stages. All of the signs and symptoms of uremia can be reversed by dialysis or "cured" by a kidney transplant.

What happens when your kidneys don't work as they should?

When there is injury or disease and kidney function in both kidneys falls to below about 25% of normal for age, sex, and body size, you develop uremia. When this happens, nitrogen-containing compounds build up in your blood and tissues. Then edema—excess fluid in tissues—can be seen and felt in your legs, beneath the skin, and around your eyes, because you are not excreting as much water as you should in your urine. This causes your blood pressure to go up. Hypertension (high blood pressure) is very common in people with diabetes and in people who have uremia. (See chapter 8 on high blood pressure.)

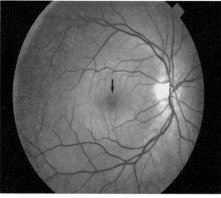

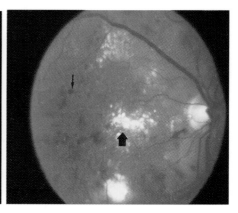

Figure 4-2a: Photograph of a normal retina. Arrow points to the normal macula.

Figure 4-2b: Retinal photograph of a patient with nonproliferative diabetic retinopathy. Large arrow indicates leakage into the central portion of the retina (macula) resulting in swelling. Small arrow indicates dot hemorrhages.

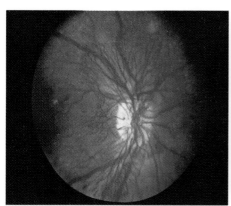

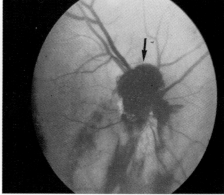

Figure 4-3: Photograph shows massive growth of new blood vessels overlying the optic nerve in a patient with proliferative diabetic retinopathy.

Figure 4-4: Arrow points to a hemorrhage overlying the optic nerve in a patient with proliferative diabetic retinopathy.

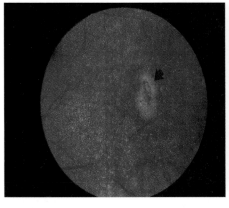

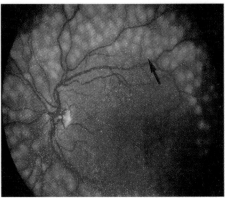

Figure 4-5: Arrow points to location of laser treatment of abnormal blood vessels (proliferation).

Figure 4-6: Wide-angle photograph of the retina. The arrow points to typical laser treatment spots involving the peripheral retinal tissue.

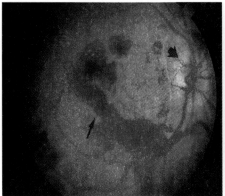

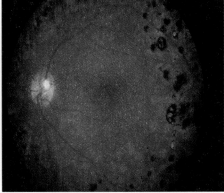

Figure 4-7a: Small arrow indicates hemorrhage overlying the retina. Large arrow points to growth of new blood vessels on the surface of the optic nerve.

Figure 4-7b: Same eye following vitrectomy surgery. The fluid in the eye is now clear, and the new blood vessels have been treated or removed.

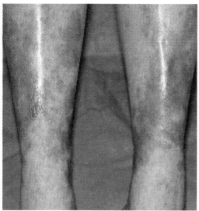

Necrobiosis lipoidica
diabetacorum (NLD)

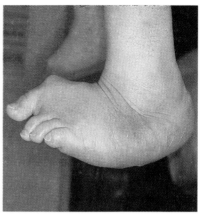

Rocker bottom foot with
Charcot's joint

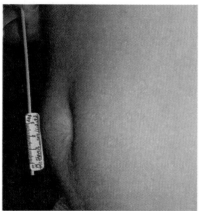

Lipoatrophy due to insulin
injections

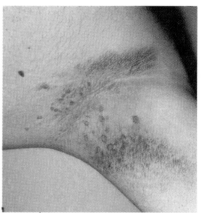

Acanthosis nigricans and
skin tags

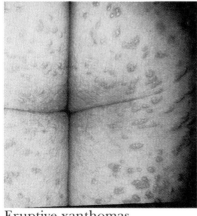

Eruptive xanthomas

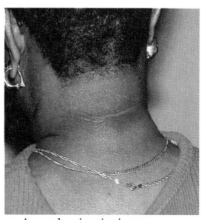

Acanthosis nigricans

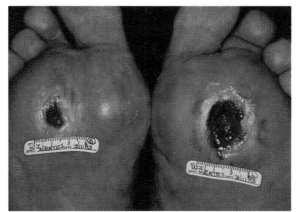

Bilateral foot ulcers in patient with
normal blood flow

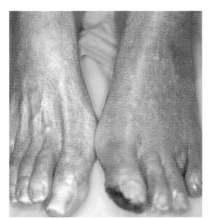

Redness of the skin and
ischemic toe ulcer

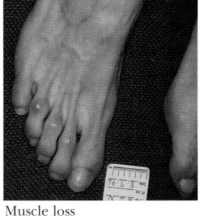

Muscle loss

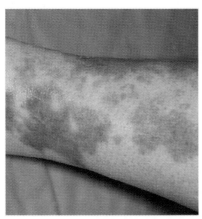

Necrobiosis diabetacorum

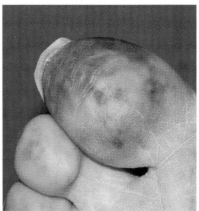

"Baked Potato" toe

What can you do to slow or prevent diabetic nephropathy?

The way you can prevent or slow kidney damage is to control high blood pressure; eat a balanced diet that is lower in fats, cholesterol, and protein; and maintain near-normal blood glucose levels.

How does controlling hypertension help?

Early detection and treatment of hypertension slows the damage to the kidneys remarkably. The single greatest technique in controlling diabetic kidney complications is to decrease high blood pressure. Hypertension (defined as blood pressure higher than 140/85 mmHg) contributes to continuing loss of kidney function. It is widely felt that people with diabetes who have microalbuminuria or proteinuria should be treated with certain blood pressure–lowering medications, particularly with an ACE inhibitor, even when they do not have hypertension. Regular testing of blood pressure protects against silent yet dangerous hypertension. At every stage of diabetic kidney disease, having normal blood pressure not only is advisable, but is the mainstay of successful therapy.

How does diet help?

Restricting dietary protein improves the condition of uremic patients and may slow the progression of renal insufficiency. Current practice limits protein intake to 40–60 g of protein a day. Lowering protein intake from typically excessive amounts to recommended amounts may be helpful in the microalbuminuria stage.

It is equally important to have a diet low in saturated fats and cholesterol. You may need to adjust your diet to unsaturated fats and to take blood cholesterol–lowering medication. This is appropriate at every stage of diabetic nephropathy. A dietitian can offer skilled advice in dealing with multiple restrictions.

How does good blood glucose control help?

Reaching and maintaining normal blood glucose levels is an effective strategy for preventing and slowing kidney complications for people with type 1 and type 2 diabetes. Of 1,441 participants in the Diabetes Control and Complications Trial (DCCT) who had type 1 diabetes, intensive control of blood glucose significantly reduced both the development and progression of early diabetic kidney disease.

What else can harm your kidneys?

High blood pressure can harm your kidneys, which is why lowering high blood pressure is one of the most important treatments for nephropathy.

Your kidneys may be injured by many drugs that you can buy over the counter, such as ibuprofen (Advil, Motrin, and others) and naproxen (Aleve), antibiotics such as cisplatin, and psychiatric medications such as lithium. There are also more than 20 other prescription nonsteroidal anti-inflammatory drugs that will damage your kidneys. If you already have reduced kidney function, the risk of damage from these drugs is greater. If you don't know whether a drug you're going to take will harm your kidneys, ask your physician and pharmacist. You and your physician must weigh the potential harm against the potential benefit of any of these drugs. Fortunately, there are safer substitutes for most of these drugs.

When the dye used for X-ray studies such as coronary angiograms or intravenous pyelograms (IVPs, which evaluate the structure of the kidneys) is injected into your vein or artery, it carries a risk of kidney failure in a few days. This condition is usually reversible but sometimes requires dialysis. If dyes must be used—for example, before urgent coronary artery bypass surgery—fluids given intravenously before and after the procedure and certain drugs, theophylline plus allopurinol, may decrease the likelihood of acute renal failure.

Finally, one thing inside your body can harm your kidneys. A neurogenic bladder—one that cannot empty urine normally—can make urine back up to the kidneys and cause damage. Infection is common in people with a neurogenic bladder. (See chapter 12 on autonomic neuropathy.)

What should you do if ESRD happens to you?

Until its later stages, renal disease in diabetes is silent. Other conditions that get worse as renal function declines divert your attention from ESRD. You may become sleepless, apprehensive, and depressed when you realize that you are faced with what seems to be an unending maze of doctors, procedures, and complaints in multiple organ systems. Medical expenses may strain family budgets. At this point, a medical team captain serving as patient advocate, physician coordinator, and friendly advisor can make the difference for you.

What is the treatment for ESRD?

ESRD is treated by repeated dialysis or by a kidney transplant.

What is dialysis?

Dialysis is a process for removing the waste products that have accumulated in the blood because of faulty or absent kidney function. They are extracted into a rinsing fluid called *dialysate*. Dialysate cleanses your blood in a machine (an artificial kidney) by a process called *hemodialysis*. There must be a connection to a blood vessel (vascular access), usually in your forearm, permitting blood to flow to and from the artificial kidney. Typically, hemodialysis is performed three times a week for 4–6 hours each time.

Another form of dialysis, called *peritoneal dialysis*, removes wastes from the blood in small blood vessels within the peritoneal membrane lining your abdominal cavity. After the physician creates a "permanent" access to this area, dialysate can be put into and drained from the abdomen at regular intervals. Continuous ambulatory peritoneal dialysis (CAPD) is the most common of this type of dialysis. During CAPD, approximately 2 liters of dialysate are infused and drained every 4–6 hours by the patient. You do not have to go to the hospital or clinic for this.

For the large majority of people with diabetes—more than 80%—who develop ESRD in the U.S., hemodialysis is the therapy. Approximately 12% of the others with ESRD will be treated with peritoneal dialysis, and the remaining 8% will receive a kidney transplant.

Peritoneal dialysis, which is relatively new, and is performed at home by trained, motivated patients, permits the longest survival and best rehabilitation of any dialysis-based therapy for diabetic ESRD. The advantages of CAPD are freedom from a machine, performance at home, rapid training, minimal cardiovascular stress, and avoidance of the need (as with hemodialysis) for an anti-clotting drug called heparin. Although some physicians call CAPD a first choice treatment for ESRD patients with diabetes, you and your physician should weigh the pros and cons of each therapeutic option before deciding what is best for you (Table 9-1). The disadvantages of CAPD are the need to pay constant attention to fluid exchange, being at constant risk of peritonitis (infection of the lining of the abdomen) that requires hospitaliza-tion, and running out of abdominal area to use.

Dialysis is not likely to give you the same long-term results as a kidney transplant. Indeed, current statistics show that about half of the people with diabetes who start on hemodialysis die within 2 years. Often this is from a heart attack because many of these patients also have hypertension and cardiovascular problems.

How does a kidney transplant help?

Successful kidney transplantation is an immediate cure for ESRD. The kidney is donated by a relative or a dead person (cadaver). It is difficult to compare kidney-trans-plant patients with dialysis patients in terms of how long they live or how well they do, because people selected for a transplant must generally be in pretty good health. Nev-ertheless, the complete renewal of life activities by the most successful transplant recipients is an impressive example of the best in modern medicine. In fact, some of the most stable transplant recipients have even had suc-cessful pregnancies.

Are there drawbacks to having a transplant?

The most serious drawback to transplant surgery is the toxic drugs that transplant recipients must take for the rest of their lives to prevent their bodies from rejecting the donated organ. The body's immune system identifies the foreign kidney as an invader and tries to kill it. Immunosuppressant drugs turn off the immune system and allow the transplanted kidney to do its work. Ironi-cally, these drugs are also strong enough to be damaging to the kidney.

More than 90% of people who get a kidney transplant survive the first year, compared to 80% on dialysis. About one in five transplant patients survive into the second decade (more than 10 years). A kidney transplant is highly preferred for newly diagnosed people with diabetes and ESRD under the age of 60.

Can a pancreas transplant cure diabetes?

Pancreas and islet transplants are the only treatments that can "cure" type 1 diabetes. A cure means that you no longer have to inject insulin or balance food, exercise, and insulin as long as the transplant works. It is easier to prevent rejection of a pancreas than rejection of an islet cell transplant, so islet transplantation remains a research procedure. For ESRD patients with type 1 diabetes, combining a pancreas transplant with a kidney transplant is now routine at most U.S. hospitals performing transplant surgery. If you are scheduled for a kidney transplant, check with your doctor about getting a pancreas as well. If it is not offered at your hospital, you may want to locate a center that does. Pancreas-kidney recipients are not only dialysis free but also insulin free. The pancreas usually comes from a cadaver and the kidney from a living donor. It is also possible to transplant one kidney and half of a pancreas from a living donor.

In one remarkable series of 995 patients with diabetes, function of both organs 1 year after the transplant was 84%. More than 90% of pancreas-kidney recipients in a worldwide registry were alive at 1 year, more than 80% had functioning kidney grafts, and more than 70% no longer required insulin. Whether having normal blood glucose levels from the pancreas transplant will stop the progression of diabetic vascular complications is now a major research question. The increasingly better prognosis for people with diabetic kidney disease shows that we are making relentless progress against a relentless disease.

Table 9-1. Choices for Uremic Patients with Diabetes

Variable	Peritoneal Dialysis	Hemodialysis	Kidney Transplant
Other serious disease	No limitation	No limitation except for hypotension	Not for patients with cardiovascular disease
Geriatric patients	No limitation	No limitation	Determined by program
Complete rehabilitation	Unlikely, persistent problems	Unlikely, persistent problems	Common as long as transplant functions
Death rate	Higher than for nondiabetic patients	Higher than for nondiabetic patients	About the same as nondiabetic patients
First-year survival	About 80%	About 80%	>90%
Survival to second decade	Undetermined because therapy relatively new	Increasing but rare	About 1 in 5
Progression of complications	Continuing attention to other conditions essential	Persistent problems	Probably reduced in type 1 diabetes by functioning pancreas + kidney. Fewer complications than in dialysis patients.
Special advantage	Can be self-performed. Avoids swings in solute and intravascular volume level.	Can be self-performed. Efficient extraction of solute and water in hours.	Cures uremia. Freedom to travel.
Disadvantage	Peritonitis. Long hours of treatment. More days hospitalized than hemodialysis or transplant.	Access point is a hazard for clotting, hemorrhage, and infection. Cyclical low blood pressure, weakness.	Cosmetic disfigurement due to drugs given to sustain transplant. Expense for medications can be stress.
Patient acceptance	Variable, usual compliance with passive tolerance for regimen. Burnout after months to years.	Variable, often do not follow dietary, diabetes, or blood pressure guidance.	Enthusiastic during periods of good renal allograft function. Exalted when pancreas proffers euglycemia. Medication noncompliance.
Bias in comparison	Delivered as first choice by enthusiasts, although emerging evidence indicates substantially higher mortality than for hemodialysis. When residual renal function lost, may be inadequate therapy.	Treatment by default. Often complicated by inattention to progressive cardiac and peripheral vascular disease. Long-term amyloidosis, malnutrition, depression.	All kidney-transplant programs preselect those patients with fewest complications. Exclusion of those older than 50 for pancreas + kidney simultaneous grafting obviously favorably prejudices outcome.
Relative cost	Has been used to circumvent initial outlay for dialysis equipment required by hemodialysis. Continuing expense of dialysate results in cost higher than a kidney transplant.	Less expensive than kidney transplant in first year; subsequent years most expensive due to professional fees and cost of supplies.	Pancreas + kidney engraftment most expensive. After first year, kidney transplant—alone—lowest cost option.

What about pancreas transplants alone for people with diabetes?

These might be considered for people with brittle diabetes who have hypoglycemia unawarenes, but you don't know how you'll respond to immunosuppressant drugs.

The first pancreas transplant was done in Minnesota in 1966. A dramatic increase in the number of transplant cases occurred beginning in the 1980s with the introduction of the antirejection drug cyclosporine. Transplantation services were also reorganized in the U.S. in 1987 through the United Network for Organ Sharing (UNOS), making it easier to find and place organs. Each year, more than 5,000 hearts, livers, and kidneys are available from cadaver donors.

At this point, only 5% of pancreas transplants are single transplants. This may change because there are new drugs—tacrolimus (Prograf) and mycophenolate mofetil (CellCept)—to supplement or replace cyclosporine that have resulted in a very low rejection rate. Indeed, the combination of these three drugs has allowed many patients to be withdrawn from the cortisone steroid-type of drugs that have been a mainstay of antirejection treatment and have side effects involving the bones and skin. This improvement in immunosuppression may lead to more single pancreas transplants in the next few years.

Is an artificial pancreas an option?

It may be possible to have an artificial pancreas implanted sometime soon, just as pumps are implanted now. We already have insulin pumps, insulin algorithms, and pump diagnostic capabilities. All that is lacking is a way to measure blood glucose levels consistently. Once this meter is invented, you might have an artificial pancreas and no need for immunosuppressant drugs.

How successful are organ transplants?

UNOS maintains an organ registry, and the outcome of nearly every surgery is known. For patients who received a pancreas-kidney transplant, 85% were dialysis free at 1 year, and 80% at 3 years. These dialysis-free rates were higher than for patients with diabetes who received only a kidney transplant. The pancreas, although it may require additional surgery, helps the transplanted kidney do its work. The rejection rate at 1 year for a pancreas-kidney transplant is only 3% and for the pancreas alone is less than 10%. Thus, most recipients of a successful transplant can expect to remain insulin free for years or for the rest of their lives.

What are the side effects of immunosuppressant drugs?

Both Prograf and cyclosporine can decrease kidney function, which can be a problem for people who already have kidney damage from diabetes. In those who have good kidney function, both Prograf and cyclosporine are usually well tolerated, but other side effects of the immunosuppressant drugs also occur, including a tendency toward obesity or osteoporosis with the cortisone like drugs. Again, cortisone-like drugs are not being used as much, especially with the introduction of Prograf and CellCept. However, at this time, you have no choice but to take some immunosuppressant drug after the transplant. The side effects must be accepted as a trade-off for being insulin free and must be considered before the surgery.

Who usually gets a transplant?

The typical patient who is a candidate for a pancreas-kidney transplant has had diabetes for 15–30 years, has developed high blood pressure, and has had an increase in the blood chemical creatinine associated with kidney failure. At this point, the nephrologist (kidney specialist) should consult with the transplant surgeon and either arrange for the patient to go on the waiting list for a cadaver donor kidney transplant or screen family members to determine who is suitable to be a kidney or kidney and half-pancreas donor. The organs that come from a living relative are more likely to be accepted by the patient's body.

The timing of when to do the kidney transplant depends on both creatinine blood levels and the patient's symptoms. Chronic fatigue and a need for blood pressure medications, along with recurrent swelling or need for diuretic (water) pills, indicate that the individual will eventually need dialysis. At this point, the patient should be placed on the waiting list for a transplant, or a living-donor transplant should be arranged.

Will more transplants be done for people with diabetes in the future?

It seems likely. The quality of life for the recipient of a successful transplant is so improved as to be restored to health. Add to that the availability of organs for transplant and the fact that the cost of a transplant when spread over the years of good health afterward is not as expensive as the dialysis option. The results of ongoing research into new and better drugs or techniques to suppress the immune system will lead to transplants being an even more popular option for people with diabetes.

Eli A. Friedman, MD, and David E.R. Sutherland, MD, PhD, contributed to this chapter.

10

Peripheral Vascular Disease

Case study

HG is a 54-year-old contractor who has had ulcers on the outside of his first and fifth toes for 2 months. He has had diabetes for 15 years and says he maintains irregular control. He is overweight, and his only regular exercise is manual labor as a contractor. HG smoked one pack of cigarettes a day for 20 years, until he quit 2 years ago after a severe respiratory illness.

HG reported that 2 months ago he wore a new pair of wing-tipped loafers to a weekend wedding. Normally, he says, he cannot feel the bottom of his feet very well, but the day after the wedding, both first and fifth toes were swollen, red, and painful. He found blisters and tried to remedy the problem himself by puncturing the blisters with a needle. He applied some antibiotic ointment and Band-Aids and went to work the following day. Two days later he reported unusual fatigue and noted increasing redness of the left foot. His blood sugar, which was erratic before, was now even more difficult to control. The family doctor prescribed an antibiotic over the phone, without evaluating HG's feet. His condition improved but then deteriorated rapidly soon after the 10-day course of antibiotic was done. At this point, he saw his doctor, who found open ulcerations on the first and fifth toes on the outside of each joint. There was marked inflammation and red streaking going up the back of the foot. The physician took cultures of the ulcers, and HG was admitted to the hospital to receive intravenous antibiotics and saline dressings. His condition improved.

Further evaluation revealed that HG had pulses that could be felt in the groin (femoral pulses) and in the knee (popliteal pulses) but no foot pulses. Circulation tests using a Doppler device revealed a moderately poor blood supply to the foot. HG took another 6-week course of antibiotics, but the ulcers never healed. He became frustrated and sought a second opinion. Fortunately, he was evaluated by a vascular surgeon with expertise in diabetic peripheral vascular disease. The vascular surgeon heard that for 5 years, the patient had noticed increasing pain in the left calf after walking shorter and shorter distances. Although this was not disabling and did not interfere with his work, HG was perplexed because his right leg seemed fine. HG also complained of numbness, tingling, and hot and cold sensations in both feet. He felt these were caused by poor circulation and used various heat remedies during and after work. The vascular surgeon examined the ulcers, and a sterile metal probe went all the way into the first joint. An X ray revealed osteomyelitis (infection in the bone). (See chapter 3.)

The surgeon pointed out the diminished hair and thinning of the skin of the left foot compared with the right. Doppler signals were much stronger in the right foot. The surgeon ordered an arteriogram (an X ray using a dye) to view the blood vessels in HG's feet and legs.

Creatinine is a measure of kidney function, and a normal value is up to 1. Because the dye used in these studies can injure the kidneys, as little dye as possible is used in patients with evidence of kidney disease. HG had a creatinine of 1.5, so the arteriogram was limited to the left leg. The arteriogram revealed that the arteries to the major organs of the body, such as the heart and kidneys, showed slight signs of atherosclerosis (plaque buildup in the blood vessels). The femoral artery (groin) and popliteal arteries (knee) had impaired circulation. There was complete blockage of the arteries below the knee (anterior tibial and posterior tibial, with severe disease of the peroneal artery). However, the dorsalis pedis artery in the foot was not badly impaired; HG had good foot blood vessels.

At a family meeting, the surgeon described a bypass operation that would restore circulation from the good popliteal artery at the knee to the dorsalis pedis artery in the top of the foot. HG had received proper dressings, complete rest of the left leg and foot, and adequate antibiotics, but there was not enough circulation to heal his foot ulcer. Also, now that the ulcer penetrated into the joint and the bone was infected, another operation would be needed to remove the infected joint and bone once circulation was restored. This would save HG's toe, which the doctor stressed was very important for HG's function and well-being.

The vascular surgeon said that he worked with a team of diabetologists, infectious disease consultants, and podiatrists to provide total care to HG. The case manager assigned to HG assisted him and his family in preparing for the surgery and what was to follow, including home care and rehabilitation.

HG, now having the information he needed, accepted the risks and underwent successful bypass grafting to the dorsalis pedis artery with a vein taken from the same lower leg. The podiatrist also performed successful joint resection (removal), saving the toe. HG was discharged without needing intravenous antibiotics and was able to recuperate at home because of the care and support he received from his family.

Two months later, HG was back to working a full schedule, wearing his work boot but with an insert to protect the previously injured foot areas. He had some moderate swelling of the left foot by the end of the day, which lessened gradually over time. Because the team concentrated on rehabilitating HG totally, he now takes excellent care of himself, regulating his diabetes at home with healthy food choices, insulin, and regular exercise. The wing-tipped loafers were donated to charity, and HG now helps educate others about the essentials of foot care.

What puts you at risk of developing peripheral vascular disease?

Peripheral vascular disease (PVD) is a condition in which plaque buildup causes a narrowing of the arteries to your legs. The case study is a typical example of PVD in patients with diabetes. PVD is 20 times more common in people with diabetes than in the general population. Other risk factors are smoking, poor nutrition, lack of exercise, high blood lipid levels (including cholesterol), and poor blood glucose control. (See chapter 6 on cholesterol.) Women with diabetes are just as much at risk, and the disease is not limited to the elderly. It is a serious disease that needs to be recognized and treated. Amputation is more common in patients with PVD. Health care professionals need to learn the appropriate care to reduce the number of amputations.

How is the diagnosis of PVD different for people with diabetes?

People with diabetes are more likely to have atherosclerosis (plaque deposited in the arteries) involving the arteries between the knee and the foot (tibial/peroneal). It is not enough for your physician to check for adequate circulation by feeling a popliteal pulse.

A second major difference in the arteries of people with diabetes is that the arterial walls frequently contain extensive calcium (Mönckeberg's sclerosis), making these arteries rigid and hard. They are not blocked, but the physician will be unable to feel a pulse in them. If the physician checks ankle and arm blood pressures, these pressures become falsely high because the vessels cannot be compressed to be measured. So higher systolic pressures in the lower leg or a high ankle-to-arm (brachial) ratio does not guarantee that there is adequate circulation. People with diabetes also tend not to develop adequate blood vessel pathways around blockages, meaning that the symptoms of these patients with narrowing or blockages can be much more dramatic than those of patients who can develop channels around blockages. An alternative to taking ankle-arm pressures is to measure toe pressures, because they do not have the calcification problem, or to measure the oxygen in the skin (transcutaneous) of the feet.

Studies show that poor circulation (ischemia) was associated with 62% of cases of nonhealing ulceration and was a cause in 46% of amputations. Remember that adequate blood flow to the skin not only depends on the underlying arterial circulation but may be greatly influenced by other factors, including skin integrity, death of tissue (necrosis) from repeated mechanical trauma, tissue swelling (edema), congestive heart failure or heart conditions with low cardiac output, and uncontrolled infection. While severely poor circulation can lead to amputation, it usually takes three causes: neuropathy (nerve damage), blood vessel blockages, and a weak response to infection. You can handle these conditions with proper diabetes management, healthy eating, and regular exercise. You need to control other risk factors such as hypertension, and you need to quit smoking. You should inspect your feet and shoes daily, keep your feet clean and dry, and wear appropriate shoes. Periodic vascular examinations will identify when you need to be followed more closely, adding noninvasive testing as needed.

What are the symptoms of PVD?

Symptoms that indicate the need for vascular intervention include claudication (pain in the calves while exercising), pain at rest, night pain, and threatened tissue loss (ulceration, gangrene, or inability to heal after minor foot surgery). Claudication is the inability to walk a given distance, usually stated in the number of city blocks (one block = 75 yards), because of muscle pain or cramping due to inadequate blood supply. The location of the muscle groups involved helps your physician distinguish whether the blockage is in the arteries (inflow) or veins (outflow) (Figure 10-1). The higher up the involved muscles are, the higher the blockage is. Claudication is made worse by an incline or a faster pace, and it is almost always relieved by rest. Patients with neuropathy may lose sensation and not be able to describe claudication in the usual fashion, noting instead numbness or a dead feeling or just having to stop after a given distance. PVD must also be distinguished from nerve irritation such as arthritis, a herniated disk, or neuropathy itself. In the case study, HG's claudication was an early sign of insufficient blood flow in the affected leg. He also had neuropathy.

Intermittent claudication does not mean you are going to lose the limb, especially in its early stages. It is all right to manage it conservatively because only 10–15% of

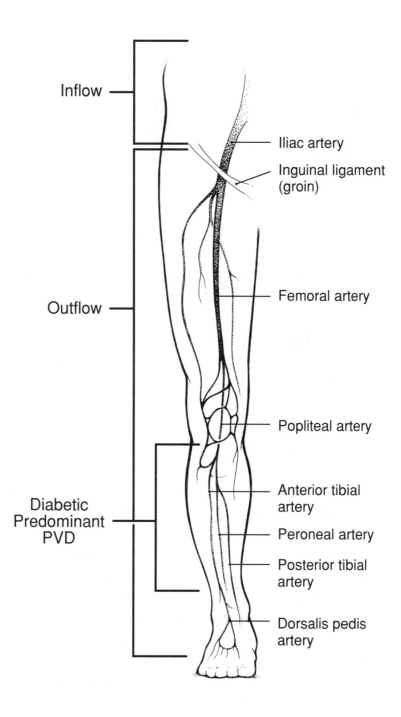

Inflow

Outflow

Diabetic
Predominant
PVD

Iliac artery

Inguinal ligament
(groin)

Femoral artery

Popliteal artery

Anterior tibial
artery

Peroneal artery

Posterior tibial
artery

Dorsalis pedis
artery

Figure 10-1. Leg arteries and veins.

patients go on to more limb-threatening symptoms. Some patients with diabetes, especially those who smoke, may progress more rapidly. Progressive claudication with walking less than 1/2 to 1 city block or that interferes with your lifestyle or work indicates a need for a vascular consultation and more serious treatment. Limb-threatening symptoms include pain at rest and tissue loss. Rest or night pain is usually distinguishable from neuropathy. Patients with impaired circulation to their legs and feet tend to describe a deep, aching pain in the foot that feels better with support of the area. Patients also tend to get up at night and hang their feet over the side of the bed or walk a few steps, which helps relieve the pain.

How is PVD diagnosed?

The physician's evaluation, judgment, and experience are still the most important means for assessing poor circulation in your legs and feet. In population-based studies, 20–30% of patients with diabetes had absent foot pulses. Also, hair growth, skin and nail texture, vein filling time, pallor of the foot when elevated, redness of the foot when it hangs down, and the appearance and temperature of the affected foot compared with the other foot are important clinical features. There are no laboratory tests that will always measure the degree of poor blood circulation or predict healing. This includes Doppler pressures, ankle-arm blood pressure ratios, toe pressures, waveform analyses, pulse-volume recordings, laser Doppler, transcutaneous (skin) oxygen determination, and magnetic resonance angioscopy (MRA). Vascular consultation and arteriography (dye studies of the arteries) are indicated when there are ulcers or wounds that fail to heal and areas that repeatedly break down despite appropriate footwear.

Blood flow can be checked by feeling arterial pulses in the feet and legs. When pulses are diminished or absent, noninvasive Doppler arterial testing should be performed to determine the differences in blood pressures from the foot to the thigh. Pressures can be compared to the opposite side and to the arm to locate potential sites of arterial blockage in the leg.

What is the best way to manage PVD?

Management requires recognition of PVD in the patient by use of arteriograms as necessary and bypass surgery to improve the blood flow through arteries to the feet (arterial revascularization).

With the help of arteriograms, more than 90% of patients with diabetes who have ischemic foot lesions (blockages in the arteries of the foot) can have the blockages surgically corrected. However, up to 50% of arteriograms done by physicians not experienced with PVD have to be repeated because of failure to carry the visualization down to the foot vessels. This adds to unnecessary costs and potential complications. MRA may replace arteriography as the procedure of choice. Because of the increased incidence of dye-related kidney complications, your physician must prepare you carefully and give you intravenous fluids before and after the procedure. Theophylline and aminophylline alone or in combination will decrease the likelihood of dye-related kidney problems.

How does the vascular surgeon decide what to do?

What the surgeon decides to do depends on your other risk factors and overall well-being. Patients who have severe dementia or mental deterioration and do not walk are not candidates for bypass surgery. Patients with extensive tissue damage or who would probably lose the limb even if the circulation were restored must be carefully evaluated as to whether they would be better served by amputation. Age by itself is not a reason not to have vascular surgery. Cost is also not a problem, because an aggressive approach to saving a limb is cost-effective. It is important for you and your health care team to assess your risk factors and other health conditions that might affect the outcome.

What needs to be done before you have bypass surgery?

Heart disease (coronary artery disease) is the leading cause of complications and death in all major vascular procedures. That is why it is so important for you to have appropriate cardiac consultation and treatment before the operation (see chapter 5). Active infection must be controlled before any vascular reconstruction. Intravenous antibiotics are needed, and your surgeon must be prepared to quickly restore circulation after the infection is controlled to prevent further ischemic damage. The choice of anesthesia is basically up to you and your team because all have been found equally safe.

What techniques might the surgeon use to restore inflow circulation?

The treatment used to correct blood vessel blockages depends on the location and extent of the blockage and your other risk factors and general health. Your vascular surgeon must be experienced with patients with diabetes and have a flexible approach. The surgeon will choose among the following procedures: endarterectomy, bypass grafting, angioplasty and laser surgery, and balloon angioplasty.

Endarterectomy

Endarterectomy is a "cleaning out" of the diseased artery. It was one of the earliest treatments but has been largely replaced by bypass grafting or balloon angioplasty. Local endarterectomy is still the procedure of choice for treatment of carotid artery disease.

Angioplasty and laser therapy

Endovascular (inside the blood vessel) techniques have been made possible by advances in technology, plastics, and optics. Space-age technology includes percutaneous transluminal angioplasty (PTA), atherectomy (rotarblade), and lasers to clear out the blood vessels. Almost all of the currently used endovascular techniques require balloon angioplasty to open the vessel wide enough for adequate blood flow. A balloon angioplasty is a procedure in which a balloon attached to a catheter (tube) is inserted into the narrowed part of the blood vessel. The balloon is then expanded to widen this part of the artery. In some cases, the surgeon will also use a stent, a tiny metal device shaped like a spring or mesh cylinder that is inserted with the balloon, expanded, and left in the blood vessel to hold it open.

It is important to understand that differences in success of endovascular procedures are based on *1)* the location of the blockage or narrowing, *2)* length of the blockage or narrowing, *3)* localized versus widespread narrowing or blockage, and *4)* composition of the plaque (calcium). Most suitable for endovascular techniques are short narrowings in arteries that are otherwise disease free. The iliac arteries (supplying blood to the lower body and legs) lend themselves to the best results, with overall initial and long-term success rates equal to those of surgery. Narrowing or blockage farther down in the lower leg or longer blockages, more widespread disease, heavily calcified plaques, and total blockage lead to less successful endovascular techniques. These are the conditions typical of a patient with diabetes and have to be evaluated. Endovascular procedures often go along with surgery when they can restore inflow and a bypass can restore circulation to a lower-leg blockage. Again a team approach helps ensure success.

What techniques might the surgeon use to restore outflow circulation?

Procedures to restore circulation in the lower leg require the use of a vein to put in place and provide a path for blood to flow around the blockage. The saphenous vein in the leg is the one most frequently used. Synthetic grafts don't work as well. People with diabetes and extensive tissue loss or gangrene of the foot need to have restoration of a pulse to the foot whenever possible for the most rapid and effective healing. Bypasses can be done all the way down to the foot arteries (Figure 10-1) and their branches to achieve this. Bypasses on legs and feet are complex and challenging procedures and are only considered when there is limb-threatening ischemia. Even 5 years after surgery, these bypass surgeries have successfully saved the limb in 87–92% of cases.

What are the drawbacks of bypass surgery?

Complication rates associated with surgery are similar to those in patients with diabetes who undergo major amputation alone, so why not take an aggressive approach to saving the leg and foot? Bypass surgery is often your best option because endovascular procedures (done inside the artery) are rarely chosen for treating blockages or narrowings of the arteries in the lower leg or below the knee of patients with diabetes. Because of the nature of diabetic lower-leg atherosclerosis, these procedures have limited success and a very high complication rate.

In conclusion

As the case study shows, in patients with diabetes, good circulation is essential to heal a foot ulcer or local foot procedure. If you come in with an infected foot ulcer, it should be immediately debrided, and you should be given intravenous antibiotics to control infection. If you do not have foot pulses or have symptoms of poor circulation, you should have an arteriogram to show the condition of your foot arteries. Preoperative evaluation of your risk factors or other conditions helps the surgeons determine the type of procedures that can be performed safely. Restoration of a pulse to the foot is crucial for healing if you have extensive tissue loss. This restoration of foot circulation allows the podiatrist or orthopedist to perform foot-saving surgery, as in the case study, to remove infected bones and prevent toe amputation.

An aggressive approach to saving the leg and foot is no more costly than major amputation. Remember that 30–50% of patients with diabetes who have experienced an amputation will have a problem in the other foot within the next few years. Your ability to live and function independently is important and is improved by an aggressive approach to saving the limb. Being treated by a team can reduce your length of stay and cost of care while maximizing your chances of keeping the limb.

This chapter was written by Gary W. Gibbons, MD, and Sheilah A. Janus.

11

Peripheral Neuropathy

Case study

Mrs. Johnson is 42 years old and has had type 1 diabetes for 20 years. She was just diagnosed with painful neuropathy in her feet. Her doctor checked the reflexes at her ankles and knees. He also checked her feet with a tuning fork and a thin wire called a monofilament, and found that Mrs. Johnson had lost some sensation in her feet. This meant that she was at risk of injuring her foot and not realizing it, which could lead to a foot ulcer. She therefore needed to take special precautions with her feet (see chapter 3).

Introduction

Peripheral neuropathy (nerve damage) is the most common long-term complication of diabetes. It affects as many as 75% of all people with diabetes. The symptoms of neuropathy range from unpleasant to severe. On average, the symptoms occur within 10 years after the onset of diabetes. Unfortunately, for many people with type 2 diabetes, the symptoms of neuropathy may be the first signs of diabetes that has actually been present for many years. Acute painful neuropathy can sometimes appear soon after you begin treating your diabetes with insulin or a sulfonylurea. As your blood glucose levels improve, the pain may go away, although the symptoms may persist for as long as 6–18 months.

Peripheral neuropathy is also called sensorimotor neuropathy, diffuse neuropathy, distal symmetric polyneuropathy (DSP) (it usually happens in both limbs at once), or painful neuropathy. When people with diabetes say that they have neuropathy, this is usually what they mean. Table 11-1 outlines various syndromes that make up peripheral neuropathy and the symptoms that can occur.

What is peripheral neuropathy?

Neuropathy is damage to the nerves. Nerves connect your brain to your spinal cord, your organs, and other parts of your body. This is called your nervous system and has several parts—the central nervous system, the peripheral nervous system, and the autonomic nervous system. The central nervous system is made up of the brain and the spinal cord. The peripheral nervous system is made up of the nerves that go farther out to areas such as your feet and toes. Because most nerve damage from diabetes occurs in the peripheral nervous system, it is called peripheral neuropathy. This type of neuropathy affects the sensory nerves, with damage to the longer nerves first. That is why the symptoms begin in the feet, and sometimes the hands, and move up. The feet are usually more severely affected. It is also called "stocking-glove" syndrome because of where the symptoms occur.

The sensorimotor nervous system includes your sensory and motor nerves. The sensory nerves send information about how things feel from the skin and internal organs to the brain. The motor nerves send information about movement from the brain to the body. For example, if you step on a sharp tack with your bare foot, the sensory nerves send a message to your brain that you are

Table 11-1. Peripheral Neuropathy and Its Symptoms

Syndrome	Symptoms
Small-fiber damage	• Loss of ability to detect temperature • "Pins and needles," tingling or burning sensation • Pain, usually worse at night • Numbness or loss of feeling • Cold extremities • Swelling of feet
Large-fiber damage	• Abnormal or unusual sensations • Loss of balance • Inability to sense position of toes and feet • Charcot's joint
Motor nerve damage	• Loss of muscle tone in hands and feet • Misshapen or deformed toes and feet • Callus formation • Open sores or ulcers on feet

in pain. The brain then sends a message back to the motor nerves telling your foot to move off the tack.

The other nervous system is the autonomic nervous system. The autonomic nervous system controls involuntary or automatic functions, such as heart rate, digestion, and bladder and sexual function. For example, the autonomic nervous system tells your heart to speed up when you are running and slow down when you stop. It helps to maintain your blood pressure whether you are standing, sitting, or lying down.

What causes peripheral neuropathy?

Neuropathy can occur from a variety of chronic illnesses such as diabetes or cancer or from exposure to toxins such as alcohol, heavy metals, or chemotherapy drugs. The causes of neuropathy are not completely known, but in diabetes, it is related to high blood glucose over a long period. The Diabetes Control and Complications Trial (DCCT) showed that intensive insulin therapy decreased the risk for neuropathy by 60% for participants in that study, who all had type 1 diabetes. The Japanese (Kumamoto) study of people with type 2 diabetes shows similar beneficial effects from good blood glucose control. For people with type 2 diabetes, high blood glucose, decreased insulin output by the pancreas, age, obesity, and duration of diabetes have all been linked to neuropathy. It is probably fair to say that neuropathy is caused not only by elevated blood glucose levels but also by a combination of genetic influences and environmental factors.

How do high blood glucose levels cause nerve damage?

There are several theories about why neuropathy occurs when blood glucose levels are high for a prolonged period. Unlike most cells in the body, nerve cells don't need insulin to pull in glucose from the bloodstream. Therefore, when blood glucose levels are above normal, the glucose level inside the nerve cells is also high. These high glucose levels may be toxic to the nerves.

Inside the cell, glucose is broken down into a substance called *sorbitol* (a sugar alcohol) by an enzyme called *aldose reductase*. Sorbitol is then converted to a form of sugar called *fructose* by another enzyme. In people with diabetes, the levels of glucose, sorbitol, and fructose are all high, which may damage nerves. One class of drugs being tested for the treatment of diabetic neuropathy is *aldose reductase inhibitors* (ARIs). ARIs prevent the breakdown of glucose into sorbitol in the cells of the nerves.

The reasons that elevated sorbitol and sugar levels damage nerves may be related to decreased *myo*-inositol levels. *myo*-Inositol is a substance that your nerves need to function normally. Glucose and *myo*-inositol molecules have similar sizes and shapes, and they compete to get into the cells. Glucose outcompetes *myo*-inositol, so when glucose levels are higher inside the cells, *myo*-inositol levels are lower. The cells are not able to function normally without adequate *myo*-inositol.

Another theory to account for nerve damage is glycation of proteins in the nerve cells. When glucose levels are elevated, glucose molecules stick to and accumulate on the protein molecules that make up new cells. (This is similar to the way glucose accumulates on the red blood cells and is measured with a glycated hemoglobin, or HbA_{1c}, test.) This buildup of glucose prevents the nerve cells from functioning normally. Their ability to send and receive signals from the brain and spinal cord may be impaired.

Another theory is based on the decreased blood flow that can occur when small blood vessels are damaged from diabetes. Decreased blood flow to the peripheral nerves may damage them over time.

People with type 1 diabetes have trouble converting some of the building blocks of fatty acids into the fatty acids that are necessary for the cells to function. As a result, there is an inadequate amount of some of the fatty acids that the cell needs.

Autoimmunity has also been suggested as a reason for nerve damage. The damaged nerves may be misread as germs and the antibodies that develop are directed toward the nerves.

What are the symptoms of neuropathy?

You can certainly have problems with nerve damage without having any symptoms, so you and your doctor may be unaware of the neuropathy. The most common symptoms of neuropathy are pain, tingling, or burning in the feet and legs or numbness of the feet. In fact, the symptoms depend on the nerves affected and the extent of the damage. Sometimes, numbness is the only sign. Diabetes can cause damage to the autonomic, sensory, and motor nerves. (For more information see chapter 17 on impotence, chapter 13 on gastrointestinal complications, chapter 5 on the heart, and chapter 12 on other autonomic neuropathies.)

How is neuropathy diagnosed?

Diabetic neuropathy can be diagnosed by signs and symptoms, after excluding other causes for them. At least once a year, your health care provider should test your reflexes and check your ability to sense vibrations with a tuning fork and your ability to sense a light touch with a monofilament.

Are there any other tests done for neuropathy?

It is not routine, but in a few confusing cases, an electrodiagnostic test of nerve function (an electromyogram [EMG] test) and a neurological examination may be done to grade the severity of sensorimotor neuropathies. These tests are generally done by a neurologist—a physician with special training in nerve diseases. Physicians more commonly use heat and cold and vibration to document the degree and extent of neuropathy.

Why is neuropathy so serious?

When sensory nerves are damaged, the most important result is loss of protective sensation. This means that because there is no pain, you may continue to walk on an injured foot. This can result in ulceration, which then can become infected, leading to gangrene and amputation. Because there is loss of sensation, it is critical to check your feet every day or have a family member do it for you. You should check not only the top of the foot but also the bottom and between the toes. For more on proper foot care, please read chapter 3. Ask your provider or nurse educator to show you the proper way to inspect your feet and how to care for them well. If you need help, do not be embarrassed to say so.

Nerves are made up of both small and large fibers. If the small fibers of the nerves are affected, you will have pain and be unable to detect heat and cold, which increases your risk for burns or frostbite. If large fibers are affected, you lose the ability to sense the position of your feet or to feel a light touch.

If the pain that results from sensorimotor neuropathy lasts for less than 6 months, it is considered acute. Pain that lasts longer than 6 months is considered chronic. With chronic painful neuropathy, the pain may eventually disappear, and your feet and hands will feel numb or always cold as the nerves become more damaged.

With large-fiber damage, your senses of balance and position are impaired, which increases your risk for falls. Some people describe this as "not being able to feel where my feet are when I walk." These people have extra difficulty walking in the dark.

When motor nerves are damaged, the muscles in the feet can become weak and eventually atrophy (degenerate). This results in the development of foot and toe deformities, such as hammertoes and claw toes.

What if your only symptom is numbness?

Actually, feet that feel numb as a result of nerve damage are more common than painful feet. If you are unable to feel a 128 tuning fork that is vibrating on your toe or you are unable to feel a monofilament wire pressing on the fleshy part of your foot, you have an insensate foot, like Mrs. Johnson in the case study. If you have any foot deformity, you will certainly benefit from custom-made foot orthoses or shoes to prevent damage to your feet. These can save your feet. See chapter 3 for detailed information on proper shoe fitting and foot care.

What is the treatment for sensorimotor neuropathy?

The treatment for sensorimotor neuropathy is based on the particular symptoms that you have. There is no cure for neuropathy, so the treatment is mostly aimed at relieving the pain and protecting your feet and hands to prevent injuries. Lowering blood glucose levels to as near normal as possible may decrease pain or other symptoms. Things you can do to care for sensorimotor neuropathies are listed in Table 11-2.

There are also medicines that can be used to relieve pain and other symptoms. Vitamins alone usually aren't effective to treat neuropathy caused by diabetes. Pain-relieving medicines that contain narcotics are generally not recommended because of side effects and the risk for addiction. Over-the-counter pain relievers and topical capsaicin 0.075% (Zostrix HP) applied to the skin may be effective. Medicines that your provider may prescribe include low doses of anticonvulsive agents (phenytoin, carbamazepine, gabapentin) and antidepressants (amitriptyline alone or with a phenothiazine, mexiletine). Many of these agents take time to work, so you need to give them a fair trial (4–6 weeks) before you decide whether they are effective. Like all medicines, these may cause side effects. Common ones are sleepiness, dry mouth, constipation, nausea, and dizziness. Taking your dose at bedtime may help. Tell your provider about these or any other side effects. Your dose may need to be adjusted. Obviously, there are many drugs to choose from, and they need to be discussed with your doctor. Sometimes, it may be helpful to see a neurologist.

Therapies used in place of or along with medications can also be helpful. Walking or gentle stretching, relaxation exercises, biofeedback, and hypnosis may help relieve your pain. Alcohol and cigarette smoking may aggravate symptoms. Elastic body stockings (available at dance or exercise stores), pantyhose, or foot cradles can help keep clothes and bedcovers away from your sensitive skin. Lamb's wool padding and specially made shoes or orthotic devices can help protect misshapen feet. Transcutaneous nerve stimulation (TENS) units are battery-operated devices that are about the size of a portable radio. TENS units provide small electrical impulses that block the pain message from getting to your brain. These devices are available only by prescription. There are also clinics in larger medical centers that specialize in pain relief. Ask your provider for a referral if you believe this would be helpful to you. Talk to your physician or nurse educator about any pain remedies you read about in newspapers or magazines. Many of these are expensive but not very effective.

Are there treatments for the pain of neuropathy?

Control of pain is one of the most difficult management issues in neuropathy. Try simple maneuvers first. Painful neuropathy can actually be brought on by beginning diabetic therapy; but it usually goes away with near normal blood glucose levels. Symptoms may persist for as long as 6 to 18 months.

Capsaicin

Burning pain may respond to capsaicin (Axain) applied topically three or four times daily. Capsaicin is extracted from chili peppers. Take care to avoid eyes and genitals,

Table 11-2. Self-care Practices for Sensorimotor Neuropathies

- Keep your blood sugar levels as close to normal as is safe for you.
- Protect your feet. You need to do what your nerves used to do for you. (See Chapter 3 for more information about foot care.)
- Give therapies a fair trial before you decide if they are working or not. Some medicines take time before they begin to work.
- Talk to your provider about any "home" or other remedies you are using or hear about. Some may be helpful, but others may actually be harmful.
- Stop cigarette smoking. Ask your provider about smoking cessation programs in your area. Nicotine delivery systems (patches, gum) are available without a prescription and may help you to be able to quit.
- Avoid alcohol because it can increase nerve damage. Ask your provider about programs in your area that can help if you believe alcohol is a problem for you.
- Keep informed and up-to-date. Take diabetes education classes to learn the best and latest techniques for protecting your health. Neuropathy is an area of ongoing research. Ask your provider periodically if there are new medicines or other therapies available. If you are interested in participating in studies of new medications, call the American Diabetes Association (ADA) at 1-800-DIABETES, look up diabetes or diabetic neuropathy on the Internet, or contact the diabetes program offered at large medical centers in your area and ask if there are any studies available.

and wear gloves when applying the creme. It is safer to cover the affected areas with plastic wrap. Initially the symptoms may get worse, followed by relief of pain in 2–3 weeks.

Nerve blocking

Lidocaine given by slow infusion has provided relief of pain for 3–21 days. This form of therapy may be most useful in self-limited forms of neuropathy. If successful, therapy can be continued with oral mexiletine. These compounds target pain caused by sensitivity of nerve endings near the surface of the skin.

Antidepressants

Several studies have shown the tricyclic antidepressants combined with the phenothiazine fluphenazine to be effective in treating painful neuropathy, with benefits unrelated to relief of depression. These drugs act by interrupting pain transmission.

Phenytoin

Diphenylhydantoin, or Dilantin, has long been used in the treatment of painful neuropathies.

Gabapentin

Gabapentin (Neurontin) is an effective anticonvulsant whose mechanism is not well understood but that holds additional promise as an analgesic agent in painful neuropathy.

Transcutaneous nerve stimulation

TENS may occasionally be helpful and certainly represents one of the more benign therapies for painful neuropathy. Care should be taken to move the electrodes around to identify sensitive areas and obtain maximal relief.

Analgesics

These are rarely of much benefit in the treatment of painful neuropathy, although they may be of some use on a short-term basis. Use of narcotics in chronic pain is generally avoided because of the risk of addiction.

In conclusion

The symptoms of both sensorimotor and autonomic neuropathy can greatly affect your overall health, lifestyle, and ability to function. You and your family need care, education, and support to deal with these neuropathies on an ongoing basis. The first steps are to learn all you can and to find a knowledgeable and compassionate health care team. The team may include physicians who are experts in diabetes, endocrinology, and/or neurology; nurse educators; a dietitian; a psychosocial expert (psychologist, social worker); and you as the leader of the team. Support groups and educational programs may also be helpful as you cope with diabetes and its complications. There is help available for you now and hope for the future as research seeks and finds new therapies.

This chatper was written by Martha M. Funnell, MS, RN, CDE; Douglas A. Greene, MD; Eva L. Feldman, MD, PhD; and Martin J. Stevens, MD.

12

The Other Neuropathies

Introduction

Peripheral neuropathy is the name for damage to motor, sensory, and autonomic nerves. Motor and sensory nerves help you move and touch the world around you. Autonomic nerves help with the activities of your body that you don't have to think about—heartbeat, breathing, food digestion. Neuropathy can further be classified as either diffuse or focal—*diffuse* meaning scattered and *focal* meaning only one or a few nerves are involved. Diffuse neuropathies develop slowly over time, and focal nerve damage tends to occur suddenly.

Damage to the motor and sensory nerves in your feet and hands is the most common type of nerve damage and the one most people are talking about when they say they have neuropathy. Damage to the autonomic nerves can affect major systems in your body, such as the heart (chapter 5), the stomach and intestines (chapter 13), or the sexual organs (chapters 17 and 18). This chapter deals with autonomic neuropathy in nerves affecting the bladder, eye, heart, sweat glands (sudomotor), and hypoglycemia awareness. Diffuse neuropathies can cause you quite a few problems. Improving blood glucose control may help reverse some of the damage done to the nerves.

Also in this chapter is a discussion of focal neuropathy, a form of autonomic neuropathy that affects single or only a few nerves in the body. The condition comes on suddenly, often with pain, does not spread from the nerves it initially affects, and gradually goes away. This form of neuropathy is uncommon,which may be in part because it is often diagnosed as something else. It may also exist along with diffuse sensorimotor neuropathy, and it is difficult to distinguish between the two.

What are the possible causes of neuropathy?

There can be many causes of neuropathy. Diabetes is not the only one. To rule out the other possible causes, your provider must consider the family history of neuropathy, vitamin B_{12} and folate deficiency, syphillis, Lyme disease, leprosy, autoimmune diseases, and toxic causes of neuropathy including alcoholism, arsenic, and a variety of drugs. Tests to confirm or rule out these other conditions will need to be done. The condition causing your neuropathy must be treated along with the neuropathy if you are to get well.

Can neuropathy be prevented?

The results of the Diabetes Control and Complications Trial (DCCT) and the Japanese study on patients with type 2 diabetes indicate that maintaining good blood glucose control can prevent or dramatically slow the development of neuropathy. Near-normal glucose levels can also help in relieving the symptoms of ongoing neuropathy. However, you may not be able to reverse extensive nerve damage, like that you find in numb feet, even with a pancreas transplant.

How is diabetic neuropathy diagnosed?

To diagnose neuropathy, your provider may gather information from five different categories. First, of course, are your symptoms. Then the provider would check your nerve function in your ability to feel touch, vibration, pain, heat, and cold. For autonomic neuropathy, it is necessary to check your body's responses to stimuli, for example, in the heart or gastrointestinal wall. There is a series of simple, noninvasive tests for detecting cardiovascular autonomic neuropathy. These tests are based on detection of heart rate and blood pressure response to a series of physical maneuvers. Specific tests are used to evaluate disordered gastrointestinal, genitourinary, and sudomotor (sweating) function and peripheral skin blood flow, all induced by autonomic diabetic neuropathy. A nerve biopsy is only done when noninvasive neurological tests do not provide a diagnosis in complicated cases. (See Table 12-1.)

Focal neuropathies are more difficult to diagnose because their symptoms are similar to those of other diseases. It is important to determine the true cause as the first step in determining the appropriate therapy.

How does autonomic neuropathy affect your bladder?

The genitourinary system includes both bladder and sex organs. The kidneys filter your blood and make urine to take away waste products. The urine goes from the kidney through the ureter into the bladder. The bladder is elastic and can expand and contract. After about 1 1/2 cups (10 oz) of urine collects in your bladder, you feel the urge to go to the bathroom. Bladder function is controlled by three different types of nerves. One transmits the signal to your brain when your bladder is full. Another causes your bladder to contract so you can pass urine. A third maintains the tone of the sphincter that opens for you to urinate and closes when you are finished. Diabetes can cause damage to all three types of nerves.

What are the symptoms of neuropathy of the bladder?

When people first begin to have this type of damage, they may urinate less often. Some people will have urgency and frequency but will pass only small amounts of urine each time. This is because the bladder does not empty completely each time. Tests for bladder function might include blood tests of your kidney function, measurement of the amount of urine left in your bladder after you urinate, or an ultrasound test of your bladder when it is full.

One of the concerns is that urine remaining in your bladder provides an excellent medium for bacteria to grow, especially if there is also glucose in the urine. This can cause a bladder or urinary tract infection (UTI). If untreated, these infections can cause kidney damage. Signs and symptoms of a bladder infection are frequent urination of small amounts, pain or burning when you urinate, being unable to urinate even though you feel the urge, and dark-colored urine. UTIs usually go away quickly with antibiotics. You need to call your provider at the first signs of an infection. If you have more than two bladder infections each year, it may be an early sign of nerve damage to your bladder. If this is true for you, talk to your provider about the need for tests of your bladder function.

What is the treatment for bladder neuropathy?

The treatment for bladder dysfunction includes both self-care activities and drug therapies. Patients with neurogenic bladder may not feel when their bladders are full. You'll have to think for your bladder. Drink plenty of flu-

Table 12-1. Symptoms of Diabetic Autonomic Neuropathies

Classification	Symptoms
Genitourinary **Bladder**	• Urinating less often • Frequent urinary tract infections • Difficulty emptying bladder completely • Weak urinary stream • Difficulty starting to urinate and dribbling afterwards; incontinence
Sexual function	*In males:* • Impotence *In females:* • Diminished vaginal lubrication • Decreased frequency of orgasm
Gastrointestinal **Stomach**	• Difficulty swallowing • Feeling full just after beginning to eat • Bloating and abdominal pain • Hypoglycemia after meals • Nausea without vomiting • Vomiting food that was eaten many hours before
Intestinal	• Diarrhea, especially at night • Constipation
Cardiovascular	• Swelling in feet • Severe dizziness on standing • Fixed heart rate • Short of breath on exertion
Counterregulation	• Loss of early warning symptoms of hypoglycemia
Sweating	• Dry hands and feet • Increased sweating on upper body • Sweating while eating certain foods
Pupils	• Delayed or absent response of pupils to darkness/light • Decreased pupil size

ids and go to the bathroom every 2 hours. You may need to press on your bladder to determine when it is full, and if necessary, push on it to start the flow of urine. Medicines to improve bladder function are available and may be effective. Drugs such as bethanechol are sometimes helpful, although, they often do not help you fully empty your bladder. The sphincter can be relaxed with terazosin or doxazosin. Self-catheterization can be useful in the case of a contracted sphincter, with generally a low risk of infection. Bladder neck surgery may help to relieve spasm of the internal sphincter. Because the external sphincter remains intact, urine will not leak out.

Does neuropathy also affect your genitals?

Autonomic neuropathy can also affect the nerves to your sexual organs. Sexual dysfunction can affect both men and women with diabetes and is discussed in chapters 17 and 18.

How does autonomic neuropathy affect your eyes?

The pupils in your eyes react to light and darkness by becoming smaller in very bright light and larger when it is dark. The response of the pupils is controlled by autonomic nerves. If these nerves are damaged, the pupils respond more slowly to darkness, so it can take longer for your eyes to adjust when you enter a dark room. You may also have more difficulty driving at night because your eyes don't respond as quickly to the lights of an oncoming car or when going from a well-lit to a darker area. You need to take precautions to ensure your safety in these situations.

How does autonomic neuropathy affect your cardiovascular system?

Autonomic nerves control your heart rate and blood pressure. In people without autonomic neuropathy, blood pressure and heart rate change slightly throughout the day in response to position (lying, sitting, and standing), stress, exercise, breathing patterns, and sleep. If the nerves to the heart and blood vessels are damaged by diabetes, the blood pressure and heart rate may respond more slowly to these factors.

If the nerves that regulate your blood pressure are damaged, blood pressure can drop quickly when you stand up and not return to a normal level as quickly as it did before the nerves were damaged. You may feel light-headed or dizzy, see black spots, or even pass out. This is called *orthostatic hypotension*. This results from blood pooling in the feet, which can lead to swelling or edema. Orthostatic hypotension is often a late development of autonomic neuropathy in patients with diabetes.

How is orthostatic hypotension diagnosed?

Because it is not unusual to feel lightheaded when you stand up too quickly, your provider needs to take your blood pressure and heart rate when you are lying and standing to diagnose orthostatic hypotension. This should be done at least once a year. If you have concerns, ask your provider to do these simple tests.

The situation can be complicated by the fact that people with advanced diabetes may have complications involving the kidney, eyes, and blood vessels, making it difficult to determine which condition is responsible for the patient's symptoms. There is also "meal-induced hypotension," in which people become dizzy soon after breakfast, occasionally after lunch, but not at all with dinner. It is difficult to relieve the morning or breakfast-related low blood pressure without aggravating the afternoon or evening high blood pressure. Loss of the daily rhythm of blood pressure control is the hallmark of autonomic neuropathy: blood pressure tends to rise at night and fall during the day. There is a risk of stroke. Your choice of low blood pressure agents is discussed below.

What is the treatment for orthostatic hypotension?

Trying to elevate blood pressure in the standing position must be balanced against preventing hypertension in the supine (lying) position. Treatment for orthostatic or postural hypotension includes better blood glucose control, an adequate salt intake to be sure that you have a large enough volume of plasma in the bloodstream, avoidance of aggravating medications such as diuretics, and safety measures to prevent falls. Raising the head of your bed on blocks (to a 30-degree angle) is helpful, and putting on waist-high elastic stockings before you get up may help prevent your blood pressure from dropping. You should put them on while lying down and not remove them until you have returned to the supine position. Clearly, they can be uncomfortable, especially in hot weather, which means that people don't like to use them. In severe cases, you may need a total body stocking or an Air Force antigravity suit.

Medications such as fludrocortisone (Florinef) may help to expand plasma volume. You must be on the alert for edema (swelling), because there is a risk of developing hypertension and congestive heart failure. Other agents (for example, phenylephrine, ephedrine, Neo-Synephrine nasal spray, beta blockers, clonidine, octreotide, and Epogen) that work more directly on the blood vessels are used to treat orthostatic hypotension. A few patients may be helped with propranolol (Inderal). Postural hypotension that occurs after eating may respond to therapy with octreotide (Sandostatin).

Does autonomic neuropathy affect your heart rate?

If the nerves that control heart rate are affected, the heart rate tends to be fast and does not change very much in response to breathing patterns, exercise, stress, or sleep.

How is neuropathy's effect on your heart rate diagnosed?

It can be diagnosed through measuring the changes in your pulse as you breathe deeply, during a Valsalva maneuver (done by bearing down as hard as you can), or before and after exercise. An electrocardiogram (ECG) and specialized computer programs may be used to do this. This effect on the heart is a serious complication because it may increase your risk for irregular heartbeat and prevent you from feeling the pain or other warning symptoms of a heart attack.

Sometimes the nerve damage prevents you from getting the usual cardiovascular benefits from aerobic exercise. If this is the case, ask your provider what kind of exercise you can do.

How does autonomic neuropathy make silent heart attacks possible?

A serious cardiac problem caused by autonomic neuropathy is the absence of heart pain (angina). You may have a so-called silent heart attack, which is a heart attack without pain. The only symptoms may be perspiration, shortness of breath, or fatigue. These symptoms call for a workup for a heart attack. One explanation for diabetes suddenly going out of control may be that a silent heart attack has occurred.

Can the diagnosis of autonomic neuropathy be serious?

For reasons that are not entirely clear, the patient with diagnosed autonomic neuropathy is susceptible to sudden death. Generally, this is seen in patients with severe autonomic dysfunction associated with neuropathy, nephropathy (kidney disease), and vascular disease, who often die as a result of kidney failure and cardiovascular disease. However, once autonomic neuropathy is diagnosed, the mortality rate can be as high as 25–50% within 5–10 years. There have been concerted efforts to identify a cause. Cardiac stress testing should be done in people in whom there is any question of heart disease, whether there is pain or not. This is especially true if the person has two or more risk factors for coronary artery disease (see chapter 5).

How are changes in the daily pattern of blood pressures connected with the risk of sudden death?

Normally, blood pressure declines at night. It has been shown that people with type 1 and type 2 diabetes and albuminuria (protein in the urine) have blunted blood pressure cycles and that their hearts may be at full throttle all the time, which may help explain the cardiovascular events that occur in this high-risk group. Damage to the vagus nerve, which supplies the lungs and heart and regulates blood pressure, may be an important factor in sudden cardiovascular death and silent heart attacks. These findings help explain the mortality risk for people with autonomic failure. When you are taking blood pressure medication and you have blunted or reversed blood pressure patterns, your doctor must be careful to consider the effects of that medication on your overnight blood pressure.

Can neuropathy cause unusual sweating?

Yes. Sweating is one way your body regulates your temperature. The autonomic sudomotor nerves control where and how much you sweat. If these nerves are damaged, sweating may be absent on your hands and feet and increased on your face and trunk. You may be unaware of the dire condition of your feet and be concerned only with the unusual increase of sweating in your upper body. The most acceptable explanation for this situation is that the body needs to get rid of heat by increasing blood flow and sweating in the upper body to compensate for the loss of peripheral autonomic nerves in the lower body.

In addition, sweating may occur when you are eating, particularly spicy foods, cheese, chocolate, red sausages, red wines, and some soft drinks. (Even people with a normal functioning autonomic nervous system may have head and face sweating when eating spicy food.)

When your sweating response is damaged, your body can't adjust the temperature. This increases your risk for heat stroke. The skin on your feet and hands can get too dry and, as part of the damage process, may not be getting the essential nutrients usually delivered by the blood vessels. Your feet may feel cold. The skin may thicken in response to decreased sweating and lubrication. The thickened skin can crack open and provide a site for bacteria and infections to start. More important is the fact that many of the new devices developed to recognize hypoglycemia rely on sweating as a symptom. These may prove useless if you have autonomic neuropathy—a little-recognized fact.

How is sudomotor nerve damage diagnosed?

Obviously, the symptoms lead to the diagnosis. Your provider can dust you with a special starch powder that turns purple when it gets wet or check your ability to feel warmth in your feet and hands.

What is the treatment for sudomotor neuropathy?

The important thing is to keep your feet and hands healthy and to use lubricating creams and oils after you bathe to keep in the moisture. You should also avoid intense heat and humidity because your body cannot regulate extreme temperatures well. Medications (propantheline hydrobromide, scopolamine patches) may help relieve unusual sweating if it is severe. Your provider may also prescribe a cholinergic blocker to decrease upper-body sweating.

Does autonomic neuropathy affect your body's response to hypoglycemia?

Yes. Autonomic nerves orchestrate your body's symptoms of and response to hypoglycemia. When there is severe autonomic damage, both the capacity to respond to hypoglycemia and the ability to counterregulate it are seriously limited. This can be life-threatening. To counterregulate low blood glucose, your body should release glucagon, epinephrine, growth hormone, cortisol, and glucose from the liver (chapter 2). If it does not, you are likely to have no symptoms of low blood glucose, or *hypoglycemia unawareness*. The autonomic symptoms of hypoglycemia usually are heart palpitations, irregular heartbeat, anxiety, and tingling around the mouth. When you have autonomic neuropathy, your symptoms—when you have any—are more likely due to the shortage of blood glucose in the brain: irritability, tiredness, confusion, forgetfulness, and loss of consciousness.

Furthermore, the epinephrine response is important to counteract hypoglycemia. When you have autonomic neuropathy and repeated episodes of hypoglycemia, this no longer happens. Because of the results of the DCCT, more people practice intensive blood glucose control, and there has been a threefold increase in hypoglycemic episodes requiring the assistance of another person. Although autonomic neuropathy may be delayed by tight control, it puts you more at risk for hypoglycemia, and you may be unaware of it happening. If the hypoglycemia becomes life-threatening, it may be necessary for you to relax your blood glucose goals. Sometimes this will restore your body's responses.

You should also be aware that the symptoms of hypoglycemia will fade over time. The longer you have had diabetes, the more likely you will have at least some degree of hypoglycemia unawareness. To catch hypoglycemia before it goes too low, check your blood glucose level, especially before you drive.

What should you do if you have hypoglycemia unawareness?

Test often and try to determine what your symptoms of hypoglycemia are. If you use insulin or a sulfonylurea drug, you and your family members and friends should know the symptoms, causes, and treatments of hypoglycemia. You need to have a source of carbohydrate with you always and an up-to-date glucagon kit handy. The kit can be prescribed by your provider, and your family and friends need to be taught how to use it. To prevent hypoglycemia from surprising you, you should check your blood glucose levels often. You may also want to wear identification jewelry stating that you have diabetes in case hypoglycemia happens when you are away from home or work.

In general, if you have bonafide hypoglycemia unawareness, to avoid life-threatening hypoglycemic episodes, you should not aim for normal glucose and HbA_{1c} levels. Often, an insulin pump will help you avoid hypoglycemia. Lispro(rapid-acting) insulin may help also.

What are focal neuropathies?

Focal neuropathy is damage to a single nerve (mononeuropathy), to nerve clusters (mononeuropathy multiplex), to nerves in the chest or abdomen (plexopathy), or to nerve roots (radiculopathy), which often mimics the pain of heart attack or appendicitis. Mononeuropathy affecting nerves to the head is called *cranial neuropathy* and can cause, for example, severe headache, drooping of one side of the face, or double vision. Mononeuropathies in areas where nerves can be trapped or compressed, such as in the wrist and palm, upper arm, elbow, and thigh, are called *entrapment neuropathies.* Carpal tunnel syndrome is an example of an entrapment neuropathy and is fairly common in people with diabetes.

How are focal neuropathies diagnosed?

First of all, focal neuropathies may be caused by many other conditions besides diabetes. It is important to determine the cause before choosing a therapy. A nerve conduction test can identify which nerves are affected. A needle electromyography helps to distinguish focal neuropathies that occur along with peripheral sensorimotor neuropathy and allow the physician to examine nerve involvement in muscles deep in the body.

What are mononeuropathies?

Mononeuropathies are lesions in a single nerve that spontaneously heal. Common mononeuropathies involve cranial, thoracic (in the chest), and peripheral nerves. Their onset is sudden and associated with pain, and they generally go away over 6–8 weeks. They must be distinguished from entrapment syndromes, which start slowly, progress, and persist without intervention, because the treatment for each is quite different.

What occurs in cranial neuropathy?

A single nerve directly from the brain is damaged. One example is when one of the nerves to the eye is involved. The symptoms include the inability to open one eyelid all of the way or at all. This is not painful but may be frightening. It usually goes away in a few days. This is one of the most common forms of cranial neuropathy.

What is entrapment neuropathy?

The entrapment neuropathies are common in people with diabetes and should be looked for in every patient with signs and symptoms of neuropathy. Common entrapments involve the median nerve in the wrist with impaired sensation in the first three fingers (carpal tunnel syndrome). Ulnar nerve entrapment in the elbow decreases sensation in the little and ring fingers. Damage to the radial nerve (in the upper arm) can cause weakness, loss of sensation on the back of the hand, and dropping of the wrist when extended. Damage to the lateral cutaneous nerve of the thigh causes thigh pain, and damage to the peroneal nerve in the knee causes foot drop. In your foot, medial and lateral plantar nerve entrapments decrease sensation on the inside and outside of the foot, respectively. Finally, tarsal tunnel syndrome may cause numbness and tingling in the foot.

What should you know about carpal tunnel syndrome?

Carpal tunnel syndrome occurs twice as frequently in people with diabetes than in healthy individuals. This may be related to repeated trauma, metabolic changes, or accumulation of fluid or edema within the confined space of the carpal tunnel. The diagnosis can be confirmed by electrophysiological study, and therapy may be a surgical release. The symptoms may spread to the whole hand and arm in carpal tunnel, and the signs may extend beyond those caused by the trapped nerve. They often involve the thumb, index finger, and one side of the middle finger. The problem is often that the true nature of your trouble goes unrecognized, and an opportunity for successful therapy is missed.

How is carpal tunnel syndrome treated?

The mainstays of nonsurgical treatment are changing how you use the wrist, special exercises, wearing a wrist splint, and taking anti-inflammatory medications. Surgical treatment consists of sectioning the volar carpal ligament and releasing the entrapped nerve.

What occurs in radiculopathy?

Radiculopathy is damage to a nerve or nerves in the trunk of the body. The primary symptom is pain in the chest (and sometimes the abdomen) that comes on suddenly and is worse at night. The pain does not seem to get worse with exertion as in coughing or exercise. Pain in the chest obviously leads your provider to look first for heart or lung problems. Once these are ruled out, other conditions that can cause similar pain are spinal disk problems, pneumonia, gastrointestinal disease, ulcers, or appendicitis. Ruling out these various conditions requires several different diagnostic procedures. Radiculopathy generally goes away within 6 months to 2 years.

What occurs in plexopathy?

Plexopathy is most commonly seen in older patients. It is uncommon and comes on suddenly. One example is the condition called femoral neuropathy, which involves damage to motor and sensory nerves in the thigh. The symptoms include pain that is sometimes worse at night in the thigh and calf. Muscle weakness can be disabling and can limit hip and knee movements. To distinguish it from sciatica, your provider may have you straighten your leg and raise it. This will be very painful if you have sciatica, but not if you have femoral neuropathy. You should recover completely, but it may last for several years before muscle strength returns to normal.

What is amyotrophy and how is it connected to neuropathy?

Amyotrophy refers to weakness or wasting of muscles. It may appear with diffuse or focal neuropathy. Muscle weakness is a helpful symptom in diagnosing neuropathy. For example, motor neuropathy can be identified by muscle weakness and wasting, pain, and twitching. It usually occurs in older individuals and affects men more frequently than women. The thigh muscles are commonly involved. It may be on one side only or on both sides of the body and is often associated with pain in the lower back or the thighs. Those affected have great difficulty rising out of a chair unaided and often "climb up" their bodies.

In the hands, one of the most striking findings is muscle weakness, especially between the thumb and the index finger. Telltale evidence that there is weakness comes from the patient's inability to hold on to objects and difficulty with fine movements such as tying laces, doing neck collar buttons, turning pages, and working at a keypad. In mononeuropathies where weakness is a prominent feature, physical therapy may be necessary to maintain good muscle tone and prevent the muscles from contracting and freezing that way.

In conclusion

Management of diabetic neuropathy encompasses a wide variety of therapies. Treatment must be individualized for you and address the symptoms and causes of your condition. (See Table 12-2.)

Aaron Vinik, MD, PhD, FCP, FACP, contributed to this chapter and the other chapters about neuropathy.

Table 12-2. Self-Care Activities for Diabetic Autonomic Neuropathies

Syndromes	Self-care
Genitourinary **Bladder dysfunction**	• Empty bladder every 2–3 hours whether you feel the urge or not. • Call your provider at the first sign of a urinary tract infection.
Sexual dysfunction	• Talk with your health care provider about your symptoms.
Gastrointestinal **Gastroparesis**	• Eat 4–6 small, mostly liquid meals each day. • Eat foods low in fat and fiber. • Take medications before eating, as recommended. • Monitor blood glucose levels often. • Give medications a fair trial.
Intestinal **Constipation**	• Increase fiber in diet. • Increase fluid intake. • Increase activity. • Use laxatives with caution.
Diarrhea	• Increase fluid intake to prevent dehydration. • Use antidiarrheals with caution.
Cardiovascular **dysfunction**	• Rise slowly after sitting or lying. After sleeping, sit on the side of the bed and let your feet dangle off the side until you adjust. • Elevate head of bed 30°. • Use elastic stockings as recommended. • Avoid strenuous and aerobic exercise or activity. • Avoid straining or lifting heavy objects. • Stop smoking.
Impaired **counterregulation**	• Test your blood glucose often, especially before and on breaks during driving on long trips. • Wear diabetes identification. • Teach family, friends, and co-workers how to recognize and treat hypoglycemia. • Keep an up-to-date glucagon kit on hand, and be sure someone around you knows how to use it.
Impaired sweating	• Avoid offending foods. • Use lotion on dry skin. • Use caution when the weather is very hot or humid.
Impaired pupil **response**	• Turn on the light when entering a dark room. • Use nightlights in dark hallways and bathroom. • Use caution when driving at night.

13

Gastrointestinal Complications

Case study

MK is a 55-year-old woman who has had type 2 diabetes for 10 years. Recently she began to experience heartburn three or four times a week and abdominal bloating and nausea, especially after eating. Her physician prescribed an antibiotic and asked her to avoid foods containing wheat. MK's symptoms did not improve.

Her physician performed a test called *esophagogastroduodenoscopy* (EGD), in which the lining of the esophagus, stomach, and small intestine is examined by looking through a camera in a small flexible tube with a light at the tip. She was given sedatives to help her relax and be comfortable during the test and a local anesthetic spray to numb her throat and prevent gagging. This examination showed moderate inflammation of the esophagus with superficial ulcers called *erosions*. Because she also had bloating and nausea, she underwent a gastric emptying test in which an egg meal was eaten and X rays were taken at regular intervals with an external camera. MK's stomach emptying was slower than normal. MK was diagnosed with gastroesophageal reflux disease (GERD) with poor stomach emptying.

She was treated with a medication that reduces the acid in the stomach for the GERD and esophageal inflammation and another medication that speeds up stomach emptying. She showed marked improvement. Regular follow-up visits were useful for adjusting dosage of medication once her symptoms went away.

Case study

MB is a 35-year-old man who has had type 1 diabetes since age 5. He has had diabetic neuropathy in his feet and hands and a history of diarrhea of five or six liquid bowel movements a day, alternating with normal bowel movements, for the past year. He consulted his physician because he was unable to control bowel movements and had leakage of stool and soiled underwear when he awoke. Because he did not have any weight loss or other signs of malabsorption, he was treated with diphenoxylate (Lomotil), an antidiarrheal agent.

The diarrhea improved to two or three bowel movements a day, but he still had stool leakage. A rectal examination showed that he had lost some feeling in the rectum. Squeeze pressures in the anal canal were almost normal. Biofeedback training played a role in helping him sense the presence of stool in the rectum and control stool leakage better.

Introduction

Your gastrointestinal (GI) tract is not just a passive biological tube containing digestive juices. Iit's a very complicated organ, and each section has its own food-processing function. The movement of your GI tract coordinates all these functions. It carries the food that gets delivered at the top through the mixing and digesting processes to the elimination of wastes at the end. This movement is controlled by a sleeve of muscles that surrounds your GI tract. The muscles are controlled by a sophisticated network of nerves. Diabetes can damage these nerves and cause GI problems.

Problems caused by diabetes can occur all along the GI tract, from the mouth to the rectum. The symptoms you experience may give you and your physician some indication of where the problem is occurring. When your stomach is affected, the condition is called *gastroparesis* (stomach paralysis). In people without autonomic neuropathy, liquids empty out of the stomach in about 10–30 minutes and solid foods in 1–2 1/2 hours. With autonomic neuropathy, both liquids and food can remain in the stomach for a longer period. When severe, gastroparesis is one of the most debilitating of all GI complications of diabetes. Other GI tract problems are esophageal disorders, diabetic diarrhea and constipation, and diseases of the pancreas.

What are the symptoms of GI complications?

The symptoms of GI problems caused by diabetes include difficulty swallowing solid or liquid food, heartburn, nausea and vomiting, abdominal pain, constipation, increased need for laxatives, diarrhea, and fecal incontinence (Figure 13-1). Many patients with gastroparesis do not have these symptoms and the only clinical feature is erratic blood glucose control or brittle diabetes.

If your symptoms are difficulty swallowing and heartburn, what condition might you have?

When food gets to your stomach, a sphincter muscle at the bottom of your esophagus closes. This prevents food and acid from coming back up into the esophagus. If muscle contractions are too weak or the sphincter does not close as it should, you will have symptoms of *gastroe-*

sophageal reflux. In gastroesophageal reflux, the contents of the stomach back up into the esophagus. You may experience a feeling that solid or liquid food stops or passes with difficulty through the throat or the chest portion of this tube. You may experience chest pain during or after eating or drinking. You may have heartburn or a burning sensation in your chest or throat after eating a meal, when lying down, or when bending over. These symptoms may awaken you from sleep. In some instances, you might only have a bad taste in your mouth and/or throat. Interestingly, two studies have shown that people with type 1 diabetes have a lower incidence of heartburn than people with type 2 and people without diabetes. This may be due to a decrease in stomach acid production in people with type 1 diabetes, whose nerve supply to the stomach acid-producing cells may be damaged.

How does your physician diagnose esophageal reflux?

An upper-GI X ray or examination with a scope can rule out esophagitis (inflammation of the esophagus) or other diseases of the mucous membranes, such as yeast infection or cancer. Chest pain means that you need to have appropriate tests done to rule out poor circulation to the heart as the cause.

What is the treatment for gastroesophageal reflux?

There are nondrug measures that can prevent reflux (heartburn), including lifestyle changes—stopping smoking, losing weight, and avoiding foods that bring on acid reflux, such as caffeine, chocolate, tomato sauce, and high-fat foods. In addition, you should not lie down for 2 hours after a meal, or you should raise your head a few inches more when you do lie down to help prevent acid reflux.

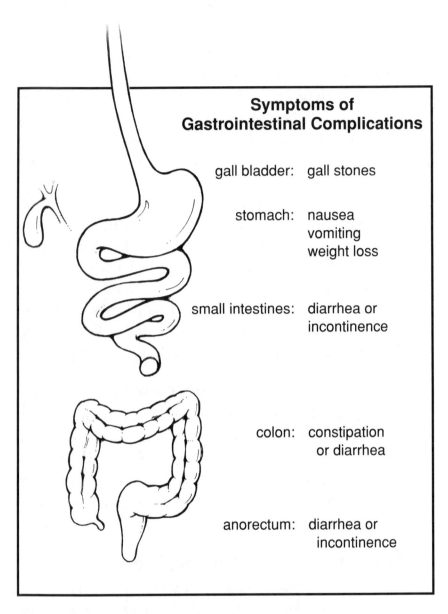

Symptoms of Gastrointestinal Complications

gall bladder:	gall stones
stomach:	nausea vomiting weight loss
small intestines:	diarrhea or incontinence
colon:	constipation or diarrhea
anorectum:	diarrhea or incontinence

Figure 13-1. Symptoms of gastrointestinal complications.

Which drugs to use for the condition depends on the severity and frequency of your symptoms and whether you have esophageal inflammation. Your options range from over-the-counter antacids to H_2 blockers, which decrease stomach acid production, to proton pump inhibitors. Proton pump inhibitors are the strongest gastricacid blockers, and they are more effective at healing esophageal ulcers caused by gastric acid. If you only have occasional symptoms of heartburn, antacids and the lifestyle changes are usually sufficient. When you have heartburn more than once a week, either an H_2 blocker, on a twice-daily regimen, or a proton pump inhibitor is the treatment of choice.

If your symptoms are nausea and vomiting, what condition might you have?

Nausea and vomiting, often accompanied by weight loss, are common symptoms of gastroparesis. These symptoms may be accompanied by abdominal bloating and a feeling of fullness after eating a meal.

Normally, your stomach's slow, steady muscular contractions break food into tiny particles. Then, your stomach pushes these liquids and solids into the small intestine. If you have gastroparesis, the grinding process of the stomach is lost. Foods are not broken up into small pieces, and they remain in the stomach too long. Episodes of nausea and vomiting may last for days or, rarely, months, or they occur in cycles. Blood glucose is probably difficult to control. You may have hypoglycemia whenever the food is not delivered to the small intestine in time to match the insulin you took before the meal.

Gastroparesis typically occurs when you also have other complications of diabetes such as retinopathy, nephropathy, and peripheral neuropathy. Other symptoms of autonomic damage are sluggish pupil responses, lack of sweating, facial sweating while eating certain foods, dizziness on standing, impotence, diminished ejaculation, and poor function of the bladder with recurring infections.

How does your physician diagnose gastroparesis?

Your physician must rule out conditions causing symptoms similar to those of delayed stomach emptying, such as chronic peptic ulcer disease, cancer, or uremia, and side effects of medications. Some of the medications that delay stomach emptying are those that are used to treat high blood pressure and depression.

To make a definite diagnosis of gastroparesis, a stomach-emptying test using solid food should be performed. During this test, your blood glucose must not be greater than 240 mg/dl because hyperglycemia by itself slows gastric emptying and the results of the test would simply reflect your high blood glucose. After you eat a radioactive meal, the level of radioactivity over your stomach is measured at different times to measure the ability of your stomach to empty food. You might also have a gastroscopy, where the doctor looks into your stomach using a scope that carries a tiny camera.

About one-third of patients with type 1 diabetes have some form of eating disorder. When this becomes significant to the extent of anorexia or bulimia (see chapter 16), then gastroparesis can develop and create a vicious cycle.

In the first 3–5 years with type 2 diabetes, you may be bothered by rapid liquid-phase gastric emptying, a condition that may slow the emptying of more solid foods from the stomach and contribute to diarrhea.

What is the treatment for gastroparesis?

Treatment for delayed stomach emptying includes changing your diet to eat small meals more often and avoiding high-fat foods and uncooked vegetables. You may try a drug that stimulates your stomach to contract and empty itself. If you have severe nausea and vomiting that lead to dehydration, you are in danger of diabetic ketoacidosis (see chapter 1) and should be hospitalized. You may need to have your stomach pumped to remove the contents quickly. Intravenous fluids should be given to correct metabolic imbalances such as ketoacidosis, uremia, hypoglycemia/hyperglycemia, or low blood potassium levels. Parenteral nutrition (a feeding tube bypassing the stomach) may be necessary if you are malnourished.

If one drug doesn't work for you, your doctor may try a different one or a combination of drugs. Sometimes a drug may be effective for weeks or months only to apparently wear off. Or the side effects may bother you too much. Your doctor may raise the dosage or try a new drug. Some people have gastroparesis for years, and then it seems to go away. Others have milder symptoms off and on all of their lives. If you have symptoms, don't give up. You may need to be referred to a specialist.

To get control of your blood glucose levels, you may need to check your blood glucose more often and when they're high, bring them down with insulin. Eating small meals throughout the day rather than a few large meals often helps. Avoid a high-fat, high-fiber diet. Avoid foods containing difficult-to-digest material, such as legumes, lentils, and citrus fruits. Undigested food may form "tumors" known as bezoars. These bezoars will worsen your symptoms of fullness, nausea, and abdominal discomfort, and they can be very difficult for a doctor to remove.

If you have heartburn, will you need an EGD?

It is not necessary for every case of heartburn to be diagnosed with an EGD. Your physician will probably treat your symptoms first. You only have an EGD in cases where the diagnosis is not clear or the first treatments have not brought any improvement.

If your symptom is diarrhea, what might the condition be?

Diarrhea is a particularly difficult problem in about 5% of people with diabetes. It can be severe and usually occurs in patients with a long history of diabetes and insulin use. Diarrhea can occur at any time and with little warning, but it commonly occurs at night. It may be associated with fecal incontinence, which is leakage of stool without the feeling of urgency to have a bowel movement.

The cause of diabetic diarrhea is not well understood. It is probably related to diabetic nerve damage (autonomic neuropathy). Neuropathy can affect the muscles that move food through the bowel and absorb fluid from the digested food. Neuropathy may also damage the anal sphincter muscles and interfere with normal sensation in the rectum. That's why people don't feel the need to have a bowel movement.

Of course, it may be caused by dietetic foods containing sorbitol (an artificial sweetener). It might be associated with conditions that disrupt absorption of nutrients, such as too much bacteria in the small intestine, celiac sprue (an unusual reaction to wheat), or more rarely, a problem with bile acid, which helps you digest fats. Very rarely, it is associated with low production of pancreatic enzymes. Certainly, this symptom is distressing enough to keep many people at home and very concerned, so the sooner treatment begins, the better.

How is diabetic diarrhea diagnosed?

If neuropathy is the cause of the diarrhea, sensation is reduced around the anus, and this can be detected with a pin. Rectal examination shows a lax sphincter that does not contract around an inserted finger. There is loss of the anal wink reflex, which is contraction of the anus in a "wink" when the skin around the anus is stroked. And there is loss of the bulbocavernosus reflex, in which the anus can be seen or felt to contract when the glans penis is squeezed between the fingers.

Before any tests are performed, you and your physician should check your diet for foods containing sorbitol (such as some sugar-free candies), excess caffeine, laxatives, and magnesium-based antacids, which are probably the most common causes of diarrhea in people with diabetes. Also, medications such as metformin can cause diarrhea.

What is the treatment for diabetic diarrhea?

Your physician may have you try a wheat gluten-free diet to see if that improves the condition or check you for food allergies. You may take a broad-spectrum antibiotic to deal with overgrowth of bacteria in the bowel. If you have small intestine bacterial overgrowth (more than 100,000 organisms per milliliter), you will be put on an antibiotic for 10 days. If that doesn't help, you may be given an antidiarrheal drug such as diphenoxylate (Lomotil).

If your condition does not improve, your physician can rule out bacteria growing in your small intestine or celiac sprue with an upper-GI endoscopy to gather bacterial cultures and to look at the small bowel lining. You may or may not need to do a 72-hour stool collection to test the fat content to check pancreatic enzyme action. You would be given pancreatic enzymes for pancreatic insufficiency in the rare event that this was the cause of your problem. In case of bile acid malabsorption (also very rare), cholestyramine, which binds bile acids, or loperamide (Imodium), which slows the transit time in the small intestine, may control diarrhea.

To treat fecal incontinence, first work on the diarrhea. It often disappears when the diarrhea improves. Many patients do not tell their physicians about the fecal incontinence, or they just call it diarrhea. It is crucial for patients and physicians to distinguish between the two conditions because specialized treatment for incontinence can help greatly.

Successful treatment for fecal incontinence includes biofeedback techniques and sphincter muscle training (also called Kegel exercises). You can be taught to squeeze and relax your sphincter muscles by a nurse educator or physical therapist. It involves squeezing as though you're trying to prevent urine or stool from coming out. Get in the habit of doing this simple exercise several times a day, say, when you're at a stop light or during TV commercials. In people with good rectal sensation, sphincter-strengthening exercises and biofeedback techniques are successful 70% of the time. The drug octreotide acetate (Sandostatin) is sometimes necessary and works well.

What is constipation?

Constipation is defined as a decrease in frequency of bowel movements to less than three per week, presence of hard stool, or need for straining. Patients with constipation may also have need to assume a contorted posture such as bending down to eliminate the stool, have a sense of incomplete evacuation, have rectal discomfort, or frequently need laxatives or enemas. Constipation is probably the most common GI complication of diabetes. It affects 25% of people with diabetes and more than 50% of those with neuropathy.

Typically, constipation comes and goes and may alternate with episodes of diarrhea. Constipation is most commonly caused either by slow colonic transit—that is, the fecal material takes too long to pass through the colon— or by some obstruction at the rectum. Obstruction can be caused by anal sphincters and/or pelvic muscles not working correctly. Pelvic muscles play an important role in normal bowel movements. If they are uncoordinated or weak, they can cause constipation. Not drinking enough water or eating enough food with fiber and not getting enough exercise can cause you to be constipated. Medications and other illnesses can also cause constipation.

What is the treatment for constipation?

Simple measures will improve constipation. Drink plenty of water during the day. Get regular exercise, which will help intestinal movement. Your bowels tend to move after a meal; take advantage of this gastrocolonic reflex by sitting on the toilet 30 minutes or so after a meal.

You should eat 20–35 grams of fiber per day, unless you have gastroparesis. Fiber is found in fruits, vegetables, legumes (beans, peas, and lentils), and whole grains. Oats, beans, peas, fresh fruits, and brown rice are great choices and should be eaten in amounts consistent with your meal plan. Food is your best source of fiber. Medications such as stool softeners or psyllium are available over the counter and may be effective when combined with other self-care measures. Excess fiber can aggravate constipation and cause gas (flatus), so you should increase the fiber in your diet gradually. Laxatives and antidiarrheal agents should be used with caution. Your body may start to depend on laxatives, and overuse of antidiarrheals can cause constipation.

If increasing dietary fiber does not relieve the constipation, a proctosigmoidoscopy enables your physician to examine the rectum and intestines with a flexible tube with a light at the end. It is less likely, but you may have a barium enema (an X ray of your intestines taken after you've been given an enema containing a soft metal called barium) or colonoscopy to evaluate your condition.

A colonoscopy enables the physician to examine the lining of your colon.

If the mucous membrane of your rectum and colon is normal, the physician may evaluate your muscles for the ability to expel stool using a simple rectal examination such as the one described above. Other tests are anorectal manometry, and evaluation of the pelvic floor muscles or the nerves supplying the muscles of the anus and rectum. If pelvic nerve and muscle function are normal, then an X ray or gamma camera test that measures the speed of movement of solid matter through the colon may be done.

If pelvic function is normal, include fiber or laxatives such as milk of magnesia in your diet. If these measures fail to help, you may need an enema program. In patients with slow colonic transit, medications that increase

Table 13-1. Prokinetic Medicines

Drug	Action	Comments
Metoclopramide (Reglan)	Decreases a gastric inhibitor (dopamine pathway) allowing the autonomic nerves to work uninhibited	Has separate effects on the brain to decrease nausea
Bethanechol (Urecholine)	Directly stimulates the autonomic nervous system pathway	May cause sweating and be confused with hypoglycemia if too large a dose is given
Erythromycin	Directly acts on muscles of GI tract like a gut hormone called motilin	An antibiotic—often loses its potency as a GI stimulator in a few months
Domperidone	Works like metoclopramide	No effects on the brain
Cisapride (Propulsid)	Directly stimulates smooth muscles in gut and stimulates local nervous system pathway	Can't use with erythromycin
Sandostatin	Decreases a gastric inhibitor (GIP, a gut hormone)	Needs to be given subcutaneously (under the skin)

colonic motility such as bisacodyl (Dulcolax), promotility agents such as cisapride (see Table 13-1), or glycerin suppositories may be helpful.

What does the symptom of chronic abdominal pain mean?

People with diabetes obviously have the same causes of abdominal pain as the general population. However, you have an increased risk of developing gallstone disease. It is probably because the gallbladder, which stores bile from the liver, does not contract as much, so bile pools in it, forms sludge, and, finally, makes stones. The pain is caused when the gallbladder attempts to push bile out and the stones get caught in the opening or too many stones are formed. Gallbladder pain may worsen after a meal or in the middle of the night and may be accompanied by nausea or vomiting.

Pain may also be caused by impaired circulation to the intestines resulting from atherosclerosis of those blood vessels. If the nerves supplying the chest and abdominal wall are affected by diabetic neuropathy, you may feel pain in the girdle area due to diabetic radiculopathy (see chapter 12.) Other causes are referral pain from the heart and gastroparesis.

In conclusion

Although there are several treatments for GI complications of diabetes, management has been only partially successful. Maintain normal glucose control and control symptoms because there are no treatments to reverse the neuropathy that plays a role in causing these GI abnormalities.

Michael Camilleri, MD; Dordaneh Maleki, MD; and Jeffrey L. Barnett, MD, contributed to this chapter.

14

Infection and Diabetes

Introduction

Infectious diseases can be caused by a large variety of microorganisms (microscopic organisms), including viruses, bacteria, fungi, and parasites. People with diabetes will get the same infections as everyone else, but certain infections tend to occur more frequently or are more severe in people with diabetes. This chapter explains how and why infections may present a special problem for you. Important aspects of the immune system (your body's system of defense against disease), the relation of blood glucose levels to infections, and the more common types of infections that occur in people with diabetes are discussed.

How does your immune system deal with infections?

Our bodies are surrounded by and colonized with vast numbers of microorganisms that would like to use us as a source of food and housing. To prevent ourselves from being infected, we have developed a remarkably effective system of defenses. Infections develop only when these defenses are breached. The first lines of defense are anatomical and physiological barriers, such as our skin and the acid in our stomach. In addition, we have a complex inner system that helps recognize invading microorganisms and destroy them.

Before discussing the immune system in greater detail, it is necessary to review the definitions of some key words:

- *Antigens* are foreign substances that trigger an immune response in your body. These include microorganisms and foreign tissue.
- *Antibodies* are highly specific proteins called *immunoglobulins* that are produced by specialized cells in your body. They help the body identify and destroy antigens.
- *Humoral immunity* refers to the production of antibodies by white blood cells called B-cells. This forms the major defense against most bacteria and viruses.
- *Cell-mediated immunity* refers to defenses by white blood cells, or T-cells, that attack an antigen directly. It is the main defense against certain bacteria and most fungi. Fungus can cause infection.

What do your white blood cells do to fight infection?

White blood cells are produced in your bone marrow and circulate in the bloodstream until they are needed to fight an invading microorganism. White blood cells are divided into six different subtypes, each serving a specialized purpose. The most important of these are *neutrophils* and *lymphocytes*.

Neutrophils are responsible for engulfing invading foreign bodies, including bacteria and viruses. Some circulate at all times, but about half are stored in the bone marrow and are only released during an infection. These cells are attracted to an infected area by chemicals that are released when tissue damage occurs.

Lymphocytes are a class of white blood cells that are responsible for generating the body's immune response. There are several different types of lymphocytes, and two main types of immunity.

What are the two types of immunity that the body uses?

Humoral immunity, as mentioned above, is controlled by lymphocytes called B-cells. B-cells are produced in the bone marrow and then stored in the tonsils, spleen, lymph nodes, and other immune system tissues. When a B-cell combines with an antigen, it forms a plasma cell. These cells then manufacture antibodies specifically targeted against that antigen. The antibodies are released into the bloodstream and search out and destroy the antigens.

Cell-mediated immunity is run by lymphocytes called T-cells, which are produced in the thymus gland. Unlike B-cells, T-cells require direct contact with an antigen. When a T-cell binds with an antigen, it produces chemicals that attract other white blood cells, such as neutrophils. These cells destroy the microorganism.

What are the symptoms of infection?

When an organism such as a bacteria or virus enters your body, it triggers a series of events designed to fight the invasion. This process produces many of the classic signs and symptoms of inflammation, such as pain, tenderness, redness, warmth, and swelling. Pain is caused by chemicals produced by the body to attract white blood cells, by the release of toxins from the invading germ, and by the destruction of the tissue under attack. These chemicals and toxins are also responsible for the heat associated with an infection. As more chemicals are released, the small blood vessel (capillary) beds near the infection dilate (expand) to allow more white blood cells to enter the infected area. This increase in blood supply causes the warmth and redness that is associated with an infection.

As the infection progresses, a thick, cloudy fluid called *pus* may form. This is made up of white blood cells, germs, tissue debris, and fluid from the blood vessels. Unlike the clear yellow drainage in many uninfected wounds, the presence of pus should be taken as evidence of an infection. As pus accumulates, it may cause a swelling called an *abscess*.

How are infections and blood glucose control connected?

The relationship between blood glucose control and infection is twofold. Poor blood glucose control over long periods appears to increase your risk for developing certain infections. When severe hyperglycemia (high blood glucose) leads to ketoacidosis, the likelihood of developing a serious infection is even greater (see chapter 1). In addition, the blood glucose level can rise dramatically when the body is under stress, such as when it is fighting an infection. Among the responses to stress are increases in the secretion of various hormones, including cortisol and glucagon (see chapters 1 and 2). These, in turn, increase the release of glucose from the liver, where it is stored and processed, so the blood glucose level goes even higher. Reducing excessive hyperglycemia (high blood glucose) is important in treating infections in people with diabetes.

Does insulin help you deal with infections?

Insulin helps lower blood glucose. When patients who use insulin are admitted to the hospital for treatment of a severe illness, they may require increased insulin doses to manage their blood glucose levels. High blood glucose levels impair the white cells' ability to digest and kill bacteria. Patients with type 2 diabetes who do not use insulin may temporarily need insulin to reduce their hyperglycemia, but once the infection or stress is under control, insulin therapy is usually no longer required.

Are people with diabetes more likely to have immune problems?

The reasons that people with diabetes are at a higher risk for developing certain infections than individuals without diabetes are not entirely clear. At least three factors are important. First, your immune system's production and use of many key infection-fighting components, such as white blood cells and antibodies, is impaired. Several defects in the infection-fighting ability of neutrophils in patients with diabetes have been discovered. Second, there are physiological and anatomical complications of diabetes, including both large and small blood vessel disease, that hinder your body's ability to deliver these anti-infection substances. The third factor resides not in your immune system but in your ability to sense the infection. Neurological damage may make you unable to sense changes associated with an ongoing infection. By the time you notice the signs and symptoms of inflammation, the infection can be quite severe.

What is the difference between normal and abnormal microorganisms that can cause infections?

Bacteria and fungi that are routinely found on certain parts of your body are called *normal flora*. Areas where these organisms grow in colonies include the skin, mouth, and intestinal tract. These organisms actually help prevent infection by other stronger microorganisms. The normal flora, like other microorganisms, can also cause infections. This may occur by overgrowth at a site where they are normally found (for example, oral thrush caused by overgrowth of a common yeastlike fungus called *Candida*) or by invading a site where they are not normally found (for example, skin bacteria infecting bone at the base of an open foot ulcer). Infections, unlike normal colony growth, are characterized by the presence of pus or by the signs of inflammation. Diabetes appears to put you more at risk for infections with organisms that rarely cause infections in people who do not have diabetes.

How are the different types of infection diagnosed?

Many different microorganisms can cause infection, but bacteria are the most important. Although there are numerous varieties of these microscopic organisms, only about a dozen are relatively common. For clinical purposes, we classify bacteria by several characteristics. Two of the most useful are *1*) whether the bacteria need oxygen (aerobic) or do not need oxygen (anaerobic) to grow and *2*) whether they appear purple (gram-positive) or pink (gram-negative) on slides containing specially stained smears of body specimens. These classifications help predict the course the infection is likely to take and the most appropriate antibiotics to use for treatment. The specific organism causing an infection is identified by culturing (growing in the lab) a specimen from the affected area—for example, urine, pus, or mucus. The most frequent bacterial types causing infections in patients with diabetes are aerobic gram-positive organisms, specifically a bacteria type of germ called Staphylococcus. Aerobic gram-negative organisms are the most common in urinary tract infections. Anaerobic organisms (both gram-positive and gram-negative) are usually found with other bacteria in deep soft-tissue infections. They are often associated with a foul odor. Each antibiotic acts against a specific group of organisms. Organisms that grow on the cultures can be tested against various antibiotics to determine how susceptible they are to each one.

Are any infections more common in people with diabetes?

People with diabetes are more likely to develop several specific types of infections. Foot ulcers are common and dangerous. For detailed information about foot ulcers, see chapter 3. In this section, we describe those infections that are most common or best studied—urinary tract infections, lower-leg infections, foot ulcers, malignant external otitis (an external ear infection), rhinocerebral mucormycosis (a fungal sinus infection), and fungal nail infections. For common skin infections, such as yeast infections, that are associated with diabetes, see chapter 15.

What type of urinary tract infections might you be more likely to develop?

You are more likely to develop infections in the urinary tract called *bacteriuria*, *cystitis*, or *pyelonephritis*.

Bacteriuria

Urine is normally sterile (free from microorganisms, or at most contains small numbers of bacteria. Infections of the urinary tract (bladder and kidney) are, however, probably the most common type of infection in people with diabetes. The term *bacteriuria* means a high number—100,000 per milliliter or greater—of bacteria present in the urine, as detected by a culture. This condition is more common in people with diabetes, especially women. Factors that further increase your chance of developing bacteriuria include being elderly, having abnormalities of your genital or urinary structures (such as an enlarged prostate gland), or having a long duration (greater than 10–15 years) of diabetes.

Bacteriuria may be *asymptomatic*, meaning it causes no symptoms, discomfort, or disease. Its importance is that it makes you more likely to develop an infection of the bladder (cystitis) or the kidneys (pyelonephritis). Asymptomatic bacteriuria usually does not require antibiotic therapy, except in people who have a bladder dysfunction or an obstruction of urinary flow or those who are pregnant, have immune system problems, or are scheduled to undergo an invasive procedure on the urinary tract, such as bladder catheterization. The benefit to anyone else taking antibiotics for this condition is outweighed by the potential side effects of taking the antibiotic and growth of antibiotic-resistant bacteria.

For people who have repeated urinary tract infections with symptoms, long-term daily doses of antibiotics help prevent bacteriuria, but reinfection occurs quickly when they are discontinued. Many different antibiotics can be used for therapy and prevention. The choice depends on the organisms that are likely to be causing the infection, the site of the infection, the frequency of the side effects, the cost of the drugs, the patient's preferences, and other factors.

Cystitis

When bacteriuria causes symptoms of bladder inflammation, you have cystitis. Symptoms of acute (sudden-onset) cystitis include pain or burning on urination, increased frequency of urination, pain over the bladder (above the pubic area), and sometimes fever. Your urine may be cloudy, have a foul odor, or even contain some blood. Most bladder infections are caused by bacteria and respond within a few days to oral antibiotic therapy.

Antibiotics are usually given for 3–10 days. Patients with diabetes are also more likely to have urinary tract infections caused by fungi, which require special, antifungal agents. Fungi can occasionally form a large mass called a *fungus ball*. These can occur anywhere in the urinary tract and may require surgical removal. Rarely, patients develop a severe form of bladder infection that is characterized by air in the bladder wall and is called *emphysematous cystitis*. This usually requires hospitalization and possibly surgery.

Pyelonephritis

Infected urine from the bladder can go up the ureters (the tubes connecting the bladder to the kidneys) to cause an infection of the kidneys called *pyelonephritis*. Acute pyelonephritis is typically characterized by fever, chills, nausea, vomiting, and severe side or upper-back pain. These symptoms may occur at the same time as, or soon after, symptoms of cystitis.

Patients with pyelonephritis may be treated on an outpatient basis if they are not experiencing severe symptoms such as high fever, severe high blood glucose levels, or vomiting. If they do have these symptoms, hospitalization with intravenous therapy is needed for a few days. The total duration of antibiotic therapy is usually 2 weeks.

If your health care provider suspects that you have pyelonephritis, especially if your symptoms have persisted for several days, an abdominal X ray should be done to look for *emphysematous pyelonephritis*. This unusual but serious complication is diagnosed by the presence of gas in the kidneys. It is estimated that 70–90% of all cases of emphysematous pyelonephritis occur in patients with diabetes, perhaps because the bacteria or fungi that cause it use the abundant sugar present in their tissues to produce the gas. As with emphysematous cystitis, this infection requires immediate hospitalization. Other complications of kidney infections include infection of the tissues surrounding the kidney and death of tissue in the kidneys. After an episode of pyelonephritis has been treated, most patients should be evaluated for anatomic or functional abnormalities of the urinary tract that may make them more likely to get infections in the future. This evaluation may include an ultrasound examination of the kidneys, measurement of urinary flow, an excretory urogram (an X ray with an injection of dye), or cystoscopy (looking into the bladder with a special instrument).

Why are you more likely to have an infection in your legs or feet?

People with diabetes are more likely to develop infections of the lower limbs for several reasons. In addition to the problems with the immune system already discussed, many people who have had diabetes for 10 years or more develop complications that increase their risk of developing a foot infection. One such complication is vascular (blood vessel) disease, which reduces blood circulation to the foot. More important, however, is neurological (nerve) disease, which can lead to several types of injury. First, the loss of protective sensation often leads to traumatic or thermal (heat) injuries. Sometimes these are not noticed by the patient and may get much worse. Second, damage to the nerves controlling muscles in the foot lead to deformities, which increase the risk for skin ulcerations. Finally, disorders of the autonomic (nonvoluntary) nervous system can lead to problems with decreased sweating and cracked skin, which may allow bacteria to enter the foot. (See chapter 3 about feet, chapter 11 about peripheral neuropathy, and chapter 12 about autonomic neuropathy.)

How are foot infections diagnosed and treated?

One of the more common entry points for lower-limb infection is the foot ulcer. The feet of people with diabetes are susceptible to developing calluses, blisters, cracks, and ulcers. Once a break in the skin occurs, microorganisms can enter the deeper tissues, causing an infection.

Uninfected ulcers require careful treatment, but antibiotic therapy is usually not needed unless the ulcer becomes infected. Infection is diagnosed by how the lesion looks. A culture tells which organisms are causing the infection. Signs and symptoms of an infected foot ulcer include redness, drainage, swelling, and warmth around the wound. If you notice any of these changes, notify your health care provider immediately. Untreated infected foot ulcers may lead to deeper and more serious infections that may threaten the limb or even your life. Occasionally, an infection may progress to the point where resection (removal) of a bone or amputation of a portion of the foot or leg may be necessary. Prompt and appropriate care of ulcers, however, can usually prevent this outcome.

Antibiotic therapy for infected foot ulcers is guided by the results of cultures of the wound. Blood tests, to check glucose level and possibly the white blood cell count, may be useful. An X ray of the foot to rule out a bone infection (osteomyelitis) is usually indicated. If the infection is treated on an outpatient basis, you should be seen every 2–3 days for at least the first week to check on the progress on the infection. If the infection worsens (higher fever, more pain, progressing redness, increased pus, etc.), contact your provider immediately. Most infections begin to improve within a few days. Antibiotic therapy is typically given for about 2 weeks for soft-tissue infections and about 6 weeks or longer for bone infections.

What other treatments are used for foot ulcers?

Healing of an ulcer requires a bed of clean granulation tissue (healthy tissue that promotes healing). This allows the body to regrow healthy skin across the open ulcer. To keep the ulcer clean and free of necrotic (dead) and infected tissue, your health care provider must perform surgical debridement (tissue removal) regularly. You should not attempt to do this yourself. Proper debridement and wound care are as important as antibiotic therapy in curing a foot infection.

Many wound dressings for covering the lesion are available. A single layer of this material is cut to size and placed in the ulcer crater with tweezers.

It is also critical not to walk or stand on the infected foot and to elevate it whenever possible. The infected area should be protected until the wound is healed. If there is edema (soft-tissue swelling) in one leg, elevating it will relieve the swelling.

To help prevent an infection, your feet need daily care and attention. See chapter 3 for proper foot care.

What other infections may you be at risk of developing?

You are at risk of developing malignant external otitis, rhinocerebral mucormycosis, onychomycosis, and yeast infections.

Malignant external otitis

Malignant, or invasive, external otitis is a serious type of external ear infection that occurs almost exclusively in patients with diabetes. The name refers to the severity of infection; it is not a cancer. This infection begins in the external ear canal, then involves the soft tissue adjacent to the ear, and may eventually spread to the bone located near the ear canal. Patients with diabetes who develop this type of bacterial infection are typically older (more than 65 years old), are predominately male, and have long-standing diabetes.

Signs of malignant external otitis include severe, persistent earache, festering and sometimes foul smelling ear discharge, and possibly hearing loss. As the infection progresses, it may involve the base of the skull or even the facial nerve, which may cause drooping of facial muscles. Patients may also have systemic signs of infection, such as fever, and elevated glucose levels and white blood cell count. Diagnosis may be aided by special X-ray or nuclear medicine (scanning) procedures.

Once diagnosed, therapy includes long-term (more than 6 weeks) antibiotics. Surgical debridement of infected tissue or bone may also be necessary. Despite appropriate therapy, the infection may recur.

Rhinocerebral mucormycosis

This uncommon fungal infection that occurs in people with diabetes, especially those who have had episodes of ketoacidosis (chapter 1), involves your nasal sinuses or the palate of your mouth. The fungi that cause this infection can grow remarkably rapidly in the presence of high concentrations of glucose and in an acid environment— such as ketoacidiosis. This infection can be life-threatening and advances rapidly.

The first symptoms are usually pain in your eyes or face, followed by yellowish white or blood-tinged nasal discharge, swelling around the eyes, increased tearing, visual blurring, and sinus or nasal tenderness. Physical examination may disclose a darkening or ulceration in the nasal passages or palate, and X-ray examinations help confirm the diagnosis.

Therapy must be started early and be aggressive to prevent spread of the infection to the brain. You need surgical removal of dead and infected tissue and antifungal and antibiotic therapy.

Onychomycosis

Onychomycosis is a fungal infection of the nails, most commonly of the great toenail. It can spread to the other nails of the feet and hands. The fungus causes the nails to become rough, thickened, and yellow. Eventually, the entire nail may become soft and crumbly and may fall off. What disturbs people most is the appearance of the nail, but the infection can lead to ulceration infection of the toe itself.

Nail fungus can be treated by oral antifungal drugs. See your physician for a fungal culture and possible treatment with prescription oral drugs such as terbinafine (Lamisil) or itraconazole (Sporanox). Your physician must take a culture from the nail and the skin beneath the nail before giving you any of the newer oral antifungal agents. Several of these drugs have side effects that you should discuss with your provider. These new drugs are used for 12 weeks of therapy with a success rate of up to 80% of nails treated. However, the fungal infection frequently returns. Also, it takes a new toenail 18 to 24 months to grow out normally after the fungus has been treated.

How can you avoid infections and disease?

The most important way to prevent infections from developing is to keep your blood glucose levels as near normal as possible. The next most important measure is part of the first—eat well-balanced meals. When you don't eat enough vegetables and whole grains and you eat too much white flour and sugary foods, your body environment is acidic, which encourages microorganisms to grow.

Are there vaccines that can help you prevent infections?

Some vaccines can protect you against infections caused by viruses. As you get older, you should protect yourself from the flu virus by getting the new flu vaccine each year, unless you are allergic to eggs. Yearly vaccinations are necessary because the viruses that cause the flu change frequently. If you are 65 years or older, you should get a one-time shot that protects against 23 of the most common strains of pneumonia. In some cases, it might be necessary to get another vaccination; check with your physician to see if yours needs to be updated. Flu vaccine is about 70% effective, and the pneumonia vaccine is about 60% effective, but both are very good at reducing the risk of serious infection, complications, and death. It is also becoming more common for people to be vaccinated against hepatitis B, a disease that can damage your liver and is becoming more widespread. Babies are now routinely given this vaccine in the first days after birth.

If you travel to other countries, you can contact your local travel agent, public health department, or the Centers for Disease Control to learn which vaccinations are recommended for your protection in the countries you'll be visiting. Again, the hepatitis B vaccine is recommended, as is a tetanus shot if you haven't had one in the past 10 years. Infections can worsen more rapidly in tropical conditions, so be extra watchful for the signs and symptoms of infection, and seek medical care early.

In conclusion

Certain infections clearly occur with greater frequency or severity in people with diabetes. Although the reasons for this are not entirely understood, there appear to be many factors, and they are related to the complications of long-standing diabetes. Fortunately, many of these infections are largely preventable. The others are usually recognizable in their early, more easily treated stages. Furthermore, modern treatment, with drug therapy and surgery when needed, can cure almost all infections. You can benefit from knowing the types of infections to watch for. Then, in partnership with your health care providers, you can avoid these complications of diabetes. Other factors that may reduce your risk for infection include establishing good blood glucose control, maintaining good body hygiene, and receiving appropriate vaccinations.

Benjamin A. Lipsky, MD, and Paul D. Baker contributed to this chapter.

15

Diabetes and Skin

Introduction

It is difficult to say whether diabetes is the cause of many skin conditions, but there are certain conditions that are more common in people with diabetes. By and large, they are not serious. Still, it is important to check your skin often for color changes or damage. Changes may be as simple as dry skin or as serious as gangrene. Even the tiniest crack can be the entryway for bacteria and infection. Fungal diseases that appear in folds of skin and on your feet need sugar and moisture to grow, and they like high blood glucose levels. The damage they can do to your skin can also allow infection to begin.

The skin changes discussed in this chapter are thick skin and stiff joints, yellow skin, diabetic dermopathy, necrobiosis lipoidica diabeticorum (NLD), granuloma annulare, scleredema, diabetic blisters, eruptive xanthoma, acanthosis nigricans, vitiligo, itchy skin, and glucagonoma. Common bacterial and fungal infections and the possible effects of certain diabetes medications on your skin are also discussed.

Are you more likely to have waxy, thick skin?

People with diabetes commonly have thickening of the skin. It may relate to accelerated aging or fraying of the elastic tissue. Under the microscope, diabetic thick skin shows increased thickness, disorganization of collagen bundles (the connective tissue of the skin), and deposits of sugarlike substances. Thickening of the skin and tendons in your hands may decrease the joint mobility and limit how far you can extend your fingers, but it is painless. Decreased joint mobility may result from stiffness in the tendons and ligaments that control the joints. This is more common when blood glucose control is poor. You can check for this condition by trying to put your hand flat on a tabletop or by putting your hands together in a praying position. If you cannot straighten your fingers out completely, you may have this condition. The skin often has a yellow waxy appearance and loses some of its surface flexibility. Improving blood glucose control has been shown in some studies to help with this condition and make the skin less thick. Otherwise, there is no known treatment.

People with diabetes are also more at risk for developing a joint mobility problem called *frozen shoulder (adhesive capsulitis)*. If you have difficulty or pain raising your arm or using your shoulder, see your health care provider, because the condition is easier to treat at the beginning with physical therapy. Once the shoulder is completely "frozen," the condition must run its course, which can take a year or more.

What is Dupuytren's contracture?

When the tendons attached to the fingers become contracted, the fingers gradually become permanently bent, and you are unable to extend them. This is referred to as *Dupuytren's contracture.* It requires surgical correction.

Is yellow skin associated with diabetes?

Yellow or yellow-orange discoloration of the skin (*carotenoderma*) is caused by increased deposits of carotene in the skin. Carotene is found in most vegetables, but the yellow or orange vegetables have the greatest amount. Carotene gives a yellow color to normal skin. This is more common in people with diabetes and people who eat a lot of yellow or orange vegetables, such as carrots. It is generally harmless and requires no specific treatment. The whites of the eyes do not become yellow, as with jaundice, which is caused by liver or gallbladder disease. *Xanthochromia* is a rare condition of yellow skin on the soles of the feet. The cause is also thought to be specific foods and the liver's reduced ability to convert carotene in foods to vitamin A. It has been suggested that people with diabetes may have a yellowish tint to their skin because a product of the metabolism of glucose has a yellow hue.

Your fingernails and toenails may also become yellow. The cause, again, is not known but may be a byproduct of glucose metabolism. Some people with diabetes, especially elderly people, develop yellow nails because of peripheral vascular disease or fungus. However, about half of the cases of yellow nails in people with diabetes have no known cause. The first sign may be a brown or yellow color on the nail. Later, all the nails can turn bright yellow.

What is diabetic dermopathy?

Diabetic dermopathy refers to small, round, colored spots on the lower leg, usually found on the shins. They are more common in older men with diabetes and, in some studies, have been documented in 70% of men with diabetes over 60 years of age. They are the most common skin sign of diabetes but, on occasion may be observed in people who do not have diabetes.

Diabetic dermopathy starts as small pink spots that gradually turn brown. They are approximately the size of an eraser on the end of a pencil, and the skin may be thinned with tiny scales on top. Although the cause is unknown, trauma, especially in people with neuropathy, may lead to this condition. It is believed that the effect of high glucose levels on collagen in the skin is responsible for the brown color. The spots will disappear spontaneously; however, new individual or clusters of spots often appear nearby. No treatment is necessary.

What is necrobiosis lipoidica diabeticorum (NLD)?

Necrobiosis lipoidica diabeticorum is the name of the red-yellow spots that may appear on the lower legs of people with diabetes—usually those with type 1 diabetes. *Necrobiosis* means the breakdown of collagen in the skin, which can be observed under the microscope in samples of tissue (biopsies) from these spots. *Lipoidica* refers to the yellow color, similar to that of fat, that is seen in the center of these spots when the surface skin has thinned. *Diabeticorum* indicates that diabetes is commonly associated with the appearance of this condition. On occasion, this skin condition may appear before there are any clinical signs or symptoms of diabetes. The condition favors young adults and occurs more often in women than in men.

This condition is not common; it occurs in only 3 of every 1,000 people with diabetes each year. NLD starts with red bumps that gradually join together and enlarge. Those spots then develop a thin yellow center, the skin becomes shiny and transparent, and you can see tiny blood vessels under the surface.

The most common location of NLD is the shin (in 90% of patients), but lesions can occur on the scalp, face, arms, and body. In one in three people, the area will become an open sore or ulcer, especially if it is located on the lower leg. The ulcer results from the very thin and fragile skin over the sore. Such an ulcer should be monitored by your health care provider. The areas that ulcerate usually have lost sensation to touch and have a limited ability to sweat. (See the color section.)

The cause of this condition is unknown. Changes in small blood vessels, an immune system response, or an injury to the skin may all play contributing roles in this condition. These spots are chronic, but they disappear spontaneously in 10–20% of cases. It is common for them to return.

Your physician may treat your symptoms. If you do not have an ulcer, you may only need to protect the area by protecting your legs from being bumped by other people or objects (wearing shin pads) and turning on the light before you get up at night to walk around. Your doctor may have you apply a steroid cream and a light bandage. It is not clear whether improved blood glucose control can help. Applying topical steroid cream and covering it with an airtight bandage or injecting steroids into the dermis (second layer of the skin) may help control the formation of new thick red areas in the skin. Once the skin has thinned, use only topical moisturizing creams. Some oral medications have been used in research studies, including low-dose aspirin and the antiplatelet drug dipyridamole. Further studies are necessary to show whether routine use of these drugs is beneficial. Ulcers, of course, require prompt treatment.

Cosmetic treatment is often important to patients, especially young women. A green-based waterproof cosmetic cream may cover areas of discoloration. Seek expert advice from an experienced cosmetologist to do your "leg colors" with a green base and added color.

What is granuloma annulare?

Granuloma annulare is an inflammatory skin disease. It is characterized by ring-shaped sores that form from flesh-colored, red, or red-brown bumps. The skin in the center of these lesions may be normal or red and is flat. The most common form of this condition appears on the hands or feet of children and young adults. There are no other symptoms, and generally, the condition limits itself.

The condition may take other forms. If it spreads across the arms, neck, and trunk, it is called generalized granuloma annulare. We do not know what causes this disease. Treatment is similar to that for NLD and includes topical and injected steroids and niacinamide. This is usually a temporary condition.

What is scleredema?

Scleredema is a rare disorder of thickened skin on the back, shoulders, and neck. (It is different from the serious disorder *scleroderma,* which has a similar-sounding name.) You may not be able to see all the areas involved, but the surface skin may look like the skin of an orange. Less common areas to check for this condition include the face, upper arms, abdomen, lower back, and tongue.

In children who may or may not have diabetes, scleredema is usually preceded by streptococcal or viral infections. A few weeks later, the child may have hardened shiny skin on his or her neck, upper back, or shoulders that cannot be wrinkled or pressed together to make folds. The condition is painless, and any symptoms appear to result from the limitation of movement by the thickened skin. This disease usually heals spontaneously but can take as long as 18 months.

In people with diabetes, scleredema is a bit different. This change is more common in men who are overweight. It may involve more areas of the body. You may have decreased sensation to pain or light touch in these areas. It may be accompanied by erythema, or redness of the skin that might be misdiagnosed as treatment-resistant cellulitis. This type of scleredema is less likely to go away on its own, and there is no treatment for it.

Can you get a blister without an injury to the skin?

Yes. Although it is uncommon, people with diabetes sometimes do develop blisters without any apparent cause. In a condition called *bullosis diabeticorum*, clear blisters appear spontaneously on your forearms, fingers, feet, or toes. The blisters arise from normal skin, range in size, are painless, and usually go away in 2–4 weeks. They become dark or black as they heal. They are common in people who have loss of nerve sensation (neuropathy) and in middle-aged to elderly patients with long-standing diabetes. Other than local care, there is no specific treatment needed. Don't break the blister. Let it dry up by itself, but notify your physician about it.

What are xanthomas?

Xanthomas are skin bumps that can accompany poorly controlled blood glucose levels and high blood fat levels—high triglycerides and high cholesterol. They most often appear on the elbows, knees, buttocks, or the site of an injury. Eruptive xanthomas can appear suddenly, and the lesions are usually 4–6 mm in diameter and yellow with a red base. The bumps are firm, not tender, and it is rare for them to break or to cause an ulcer. Biopsy (tissue sample) findings indicate collections of lipids (fats) within the second layer of skin. (See the color section.)

Improving blood glucose control and lowering blood fat levels makes xanthomas disappear. Sometimes insulin is required to correct the underlying causes.

Xanthelasma palpebrarum is the name of a xanthoma on the eyelid. Xanthelasmas are the most common type of xanthoma. They may be caused by high blood fats (high cholesterol) and are a sign to your provider to check your cholesterol level. They begin as small yellow-orange bumps, grow, thicken, and can eventually cover the entire eyelid. They are more likely to occur in women than in men.

What is acanthosis nigricans?

In *acanthosis nigricans*, velvety tan to dark brown areas are seen on the sides of the neck, sides of the body, armpits, and groin. Additional possible locations include joints of the hand and fingers, elbows, and knees. This condition may be associated with obesity and type 2 diabetes with high insulin resistance. Patients with this condition frequently require high doses of insulin. Weight loss and improved blood glucose control improve the condition. Otherwise, the only treatment is topical agents such as retinoic acid and urea, if you want to improve the cosmetic appearance. (See the color section.)

What is vitiligo?

Vitiligo is a condition of patches of skin that have lost pigment and have no color. If you get a suntan, these areas do not tan. There are fungal infections that can look like vitiligo, so see your provider for a proper diagnosis. Commonly, it affects the trunk of the body, but it may also appear at openings such as the nostrils, eyes, and mouth.

Vitiligo may be an immune disorder, and there is no treatment except to cover it with makeup. It is more common in people with type 1 diabetes. (See the color section.)

Are you more likely to have itchy skin with diabetes?

You will not necessarily have itchy skin. *Pruritus* is the name for local or generalized itching. When it affects feet and legs, it may be very bothersome and cause you to scratch a great deal. This is dangerous because scratching can damage the skin. Elderly patients are usually the ones who have this problem, but it can be resolved by using moisturizing or steroid cream. The itching may be due to an irritation of sensory nerve endings. Diabetes can seriously affect your kidneys, and itchy skin may be one of the symptoms of kidney complications (see chapter 9). Uremia, or elevated levels of urea in the blood, can also cause itching. Maintaining close-to-normal blood glucose levels and kidney function may help. Over time, the condition may go away on its own. Sometimes medicine (such as Periactin) is needed.

People with diabetes are more likely to develop *herpes zoster*, or shingles, a disease involving the nerves that causes very painful itching. Improving nutrition and achieving better blood glucose control can help.

What is a glucagonoma?

A *glucagonoma* is a tumor affecting the pancreas islet cells that produce the hormone glucagon. It can cause a red or brownish red skin rash called *necrolytic migratory erythema*. These skin lesions can appear on the lower abdomen, buttocks, hands, feet, or legs. This condition is chronic and may precede the discovery of the tumor by several years. The tongue may appear smooth and bright red. Patients with this condition also have anemia, diarrhea, and weight loss. Of course, the tumor needs to be removed or treated, which will resolve the rash, but glucose given in saline has been found to treat the rash successfully.

What are some of the common skin infections associated with diabetes?

People with higher levels of glucose in their blood are more likely to have skin infections. Having some of the complications of diabetes, such as blood vessel narrowing, will also contribute to the occurrence of these infections. *Candida* (or yeast) infections, bacterial infections, and other fungal infections of the skin are discussed below.

Fungal infections are usually caused by one of two types of fungi: dermatophytes or yeasts, such as *Candida*. The areas most frequently involved are moist skin crevices in the armpit, groin, or under the breasts. Infections cause redness, scaling, itching, and sometimes skin breakdown. They are easily treated with antifungal creams and can be prevented by keeping these areas clean and dry and by controlling blood glucose levels.

Candida infections

Candida is a yeast that will infect moist areas of the skin or mucous membranes in areas such as the mouth, vagina, or rectum. *Candida* infections appear differently in various regions of the body. Inside the mouth, white, curdlike growths appear on the tongue or inner surface of the cheeks. When these are scraped, the surface often bleeds. At the corner of the mouth, yeast infections are often red and moist. The medical terms for *Candida* in this location are *angular stomatitis* and *perleche*. The skin in body folds under the arms, under the breasts, on the sides of the groin, and around the anus also provide warmth and moisture that attracts *Candida* infections. In these locations a bright red spot is often surrounded by smaller dotted spots that may have central yellow pustules. In the vagina, *Candida* infections are similar to those in the mouth, with a white curdlike appearance that will bleed when removed. Infections in the vagina and other areas of the body are often extremely itchy.

The treatment of yeast infections is aided by good blood glucose control. In the mouth, nystatin solution (an antiyeast antibiotic) may be used in a swish-and-spit technique three or four times a day for 5–7 days. Clotrimazole (another antibiotic) oral lozenges can be used daily until the condition clears up. Sometimes, *Candida* in the mouth is resistant to topical approaches, or it may extend down the throat into the esophagus. In these cases, a single oral dose of fluconazole or another similar oral antifungal drug may be used. At the corners of the mouth, topical antifungal drugs—nystatin, terbinafine, clotrimazole, miconazole, ketoconazole, or econazole—may be useful. They are generally applied once or twice a day initially and then once or twice a week after the rash has been resolved to prevent recurrences.

The corners of the mouth must be kept clean and dry. It is often useful to eat fruits and vegetables with a fork and to drink juices with a straw to prevent moisture from accumulating at the corners of the mouth.

In the body folds, it is important to control yeast infections because they can lead to secondary bacterial infections and surface breakdown of the skin. The area should be kept clean using a mild soap. After cleansing, the area should be thoroughly patted dry and an antifungal drug should be applied.

In the vaginal area, internal yeast infections are treated with over-the-counter or prescription vaginal creams or vaginal suppositories. These infections often cause a disturbing itch and may be accompanied by a vaginal discharge. Difficult cases may require oral antiyeast therapy with a single dose of fluoconazole or several days of an oral antifungal drug such as itraconazole or ketoconazole.

Cleanse the rectal area with water before using a topical antifungal agent. If stools are liquid or loosely formed, you need to eat more fiber or add bulk-forming agents to your diet.

Candidal infections often come back, so your physician may advise a preventative program of using antifungal powders applied with a cotton ball or periodic application of topical antifungal creams to prevent the infection from returning.

Bacterial infections

Bacteria can cause many different changes in the skin. The infections can involve both the outer layer of skin (epidermis) and the deeper, second layer of skin (dermis). These infections include impetigo, erythrasma, erysipelas, folliculitis, carbuncles, furuncles, cellulitis, the very rare necrotizing fasciitis and cellulitis, and abscesses. See chapter 14 for more on infections.

Impetigo

Impetigo is a yellow, honeycomb-crusted spot on a red base that is often seen on the face or hands. It may sometimes be associated with blisters. This infection involves the epidermis. It is caused by bacteria called *Staphylococcus aureus* or *Streptococcus*.

Localized impetigo is often successfully treated with antibacterials such as mupirocin (Bactroban) or bacitracin (Baciquent). If multiple spots are present, oral antibiotics are often necessary. People with bacterial infections (as well as their close personal contacts) may be carrying organisms in their nostrils, groin, or other parts of the body not involved with the skin rash. Your doctor may want to culture these areas to be sure further treatment is not necessary.

Erythrasma

This superficial bacterial infection, caused by *Corynebacterium minutissimum*, manifests as brownish, itchy patches in moist skin folds, particularly in the genital and underarm areas. Erythrasma resembles fungal skin infections, but the lesion borders are not elevated, there are no satellite lesions, and microscopic preparations do not show fungal elements. Diagnosis can usually be made by the characteristic appearance but can be confirmed by a Wood's lamp. Under ultraviolet light, the patches emit a characteristic coral-red fluorescence (glow). The condition often has no symptoms, but it may cause itching or even breakdown of the skin. If treatment is required because of symptoms, the oral antibiotic erythromycin is usually effective.

Erysipelas

Deeper infections in the second layer of skin include erysipelas. Erysipelas usually presents with hot, red, hive-like spots on one side of the face, but it may spread quickly. This infection will often make you feel ill with general malaise and fever. Prompt attention is important, and an emergency visit to your doctor at the nearest hospital is advised. Treatment usually requires intravenous antibiotics.

Carbuncles, furuncles

Diabetes appears to increase your likelihood of developing several common, as well as some uncommon, skin and skin structure infections. Bacterial infections are usually caused by *Staphylococci*, especially *Staphylococcus aureus*. Part of the reason people with diabetes are predisposed to these infections is a high rate of colonization of the nose with *Staphylococci*, which then shed onto the skin. These infections often begin in hair follicles and are thus called *folliculitis*. Larger and deeper infections are called *furuncles*, which may then progress to carbuncles. The latter lesion most often occurs on the back of the neck. These infections cause red, warm, tender ("sore as a boil") swellings of the skin, sometimes with draining pus. Mild infections may respond to antibiotic therapy alone, but more extensive lesions require surgical drainage.

Cellulitis

Another type of skin infection that appears to be more frequent or severe in people with diabetes is called *cellulitis*, which is a red and tender swelling often on the feet or legs but occasionally elsewhere. Here, the infection spreads more superficially and is most often caused by *Streptococci*. This infection usually responds promptly (within 36–48 hours) to antibiotic therapy, although it may appear to worsen in the first 24 hours. If the infection does not improve, it is important to reevaluate and look for organisms resistant to the antibiotic you are taking or for a more serious infection, such as a necrotizing fasciitis or cellulitis. Unless these infections are caught in the very early stages, intravenous antibiotics are necessary.

Necrotizing fasciitis and cellulitis

People with diabetes are more susceptible to these potentially life-threatening, subcutaneous (below the skin) soft-tissue infections. Infection causing death of soft tissue is called *necrotizing fasciitis*. Fasciitis means involvement of the skin down to the fascia, the tissue that covers the muscle. *Necrotizing cellulitis* usually involves the muscle as well. Gangrene may also develop, and it usually causes gas in tissues. Necrotizing infections are characterized by their rapid onset and spread, with tissue destruction. Clues to their presence include severe pain, development of blisters, and bleeding into the skin. They are often caused by a mixture of different types of bacterial organisms. Fortunately, these types of infection are uncommon. They are more apt to occur in patients with impaired circulation, after trauma, and in deeper infections, especially of the lower extremities, genital, or rectal areas. A particular form of necrotizing infection that involves the male genitals is called *Fournier's gangrene*. Treatment for these infections must include immediate, aggressive surgical debridement of the necrotic tissue along with broad-spectrum intravenous antibiotics.

Abscesses

An abscess is a confined area containing a collection of microorganisms (usually bacteria) and white blood cells (pus). In people with diabetes, these may occur in the area of insulin injections and are often caused by contaminated needles, syringes, or multiple-dose vials. To help prevent this problem, you should clean your injection site and the tops of any multiuse vials.

Fungal infections

Fungal infections may appear between your toes, around your groin, on the bottoms of your feet, on the palms of your hands, or on and under your nails. These infections may not be more common in people with diabetes, but scratching at a fungal infection may break down the normal skin barrier and allow bacteria to gain entry, which can lead to more serious conditions for you. The two key elements in stopping these infections are achieving good blood glucose control and limiting the moisture that builds up in skin-fold areas.

Fungal infections usually start between the fourth and fifth toes because this is where the toes are most tightly compacted. White and softened skin is the first sign of infection that gradually spreads to the other toe web spaces. It can be treated with topical over-the-counter antifungals (clotrimazole, miconazole) twice a day. Dry between your toes very well after bathing and then apply the topical antifungal. When the infection clears, use an antifungal powder daily to keep the toe webs dry. Sensible shoes and socks that breathe and don't make your feet sweat will also help prevent recurrences.

Fungal infections of the groin are more common in men. They involve the inner thighs, with a red active scaly area and central clearing, and spare the scrotum. Use topical antifungals once or twice a day for active infection and antifungal powder to help prevent recurrences. Boxer shorts can help keep the area dry. Tight-fitting clothing, overweight, and athletic activities with a lot of sweating and friction lead to frequent recurrences.

Another fungal infection involves the soles of your feet and palms of your hands. A dry powdery scale that often starts in a small area gradually spreads to the entire sole or palm surface. The dry skin often spreads around the sides of the feet, which is referred to as "moccasin-type" changes. If topical antifungal cream is not successful, you may need a short course of oral antifungal agents (terbinafine, itraconazole).

The most cosmetically disturbing fungal infection involves your fingernails and toenails. The nails become thick and yellow. This infection is most common in the large toenails but can spread to the other nails of the feet or hands. Infected nails often have dark streaks in them, too. The nail becomes thickened and dull, and the skin beneath the nail is damaged as well. Eventually, the entire nail may become soft and crumbly and may fall off.

Fungal infection of the feet or toe webs can be treated with a number of topical over-the-counter or prescription antifungal agents. If you have a resistant case or a nail infection, see your health care professional for fungal culture and possible treatment with prescription oral agents such as terbinafine (Lamisil) or itraconazole (Sporanox). Your physician must take a culture from the nail and the skin beneath the nail before giving you any of the newer oral antifungal agents. Some of these drugs have side effects that you should discuss with your provider. These new drugs are used for 12 weeks of therapy with a success rate of up to 80% of the involved nails. However, the fungal infection frequently returns. Remember that a toenail takes 18–24 months to grow out normally after the fungus has been treated.

Do diabetes medications affect your skin?

Yes. The oral diabetes medications called sulfonylureas can cause minor changes in your skin, and so can insulin.

Sulfonylureas

Common oral drugs used to control diabetes include first- and second-generation oral agents called sulfonylureas. Two are tolbutamide and chlorpropamide. Skin rashes are the most common side effect in the first few months of therapy and are seen in 1–5% of cases. The rash often looks like measles. Be careful in the sun. Hives and an allergic reaction can occur on sun-exposed skin. The measleslike rash may disappear on its own even if you continue taking the medication, but other kinds of rashes would require you to stop taking this medication.

Any alcohol that you drink may interact with chlorpropamide and cause flushing of your whole body and especially your face. Skin reactions and flushing are uncommon with the newer second-generation sulfonylureas. If you have a reaction to oral sulfonylurea drugs, there is approximately a 20% chance of your reacting to a number of related chemicals, including

- permanent hair dye (paraphenylenediamine)
- a component of sun screens called PABA (para-aminobenzoic acid)
- local anesthetic creams (benzocaine)
- some diuretic pills (hydrochlorothiazide)
- sulfonamide antibiotics

Insulin

Skin reactions to insulin are less common with newer, purer forms of insulin. Local reactions may start with burning at the injection site, followed by a hivelike reaction that may fade over hours to days. Skin reactions may be immediate or delayed. Generalized hives and even anaphylaxis (respiratory or circulatory collapse) due to insulin allergy are extremely rare.

Delayed reactions at insulin injection sites include changes in the fat under the skin. The fat may be decreased, causing little indentations on the surface (lipoatrophy), but this complication is much less common with newer purified insulins. If an insulin site is used repeatedly for years, the fat may actually increase in size, causing an elevated bump (hypertrophy). This is a very common condition, and repeatedly injecting into this area is a common cause of brittle diabetes. Darkening or thickening of the skin may also be seen at insulin injection sites.

What is special about the skin on your feet?

Your feet can be threatened by triple jeopardy—neuropathy, infection, and impaired blood supply. An ulcer can go unnoticed because of neuropathy—you can't feel it. This can be the entry point for infection. The ulcer may not heal because of inadequate blood supply to the feet. Ulcers that will not heal can lead to amputation. Keeping the skin clean, dry, and healthy by getting proper treatment early rather than late is the way to take care of your feet. Good foot care begins with the skin! (See chapter 3 on feet and chapter 14 on infection.)

Neuropathy in the foot causes loss of feeling and autonomic (flushing or sweating) response. The loss of the flushing response results in dry skin on the feet—the moisture content in the top layer of skin drops below 10%. Fungal infection can also cause dry feet. Moisture can be replaced by covering the foot with a greasy coating as soon as you get out of the bath or shower to prevent water loss (lubricants) or by using moisturizers that bind water to the skin surface (humectants). Lubricating creams or cold creams include Vaseline, Keri lotion, Lubriderm, and many others. They frequently contain urea (Uremol, Ultramide) or lactic acid (Lachydrin, Lacticare). Creams or lotions that bind water to the surface should be applied after bathing while the skin is still damp. Do not put any lotion or cream between your toes. Put on clean socks every day and change your shoes, when it is possible or convenient, after wearing them for four hours. Taking care of your feet every day is a good investment of your time and energy.

R. Gary Sibbald, MD, contributed to this chapter.

16

Psychosocial Complications

Introduction

Diabetes can be a heck of a disease. Even if your blood glucose control is good and you haven't developed any long-term complications, living with diabetes is no fun. There are no vacations: diabetes is a 24-hour-a-day, 365-day-a-year proposition. Add to that the fact that diabetes affects every aspect of your life, forces you to stick yourself countless times a day, and makes you deprive yourself of foods you crave. And that's not all. If you succeed in keeping your blood glucose levels close to normal, your risk of going too low (hypoglycemia) goes up, and often so does your weight. To top it off, you must live with the fact that there are no guarantees when it comes to diabetes. You can do everything right and still get a blood glucose reading you can't explain.

It's no wonder that a condition we call "diabetes overwhelmus" is so common. Many people are simply overwhelmed by the daily demands of their diabetes treatment. Diabetes overwhelmus may not be an official term, but it is a serious problem. People who suffer from it tell us they are often caught in a negative spiral. Feeling overwhelmed, they find it terribly hard to maintain good self-care, which leads to worsened blood glucose control, which makes their diabetes overwhelmus even worse.

In this chapter, we tell you about the various forms diabetes overwhelmus can take, how common each one is among people with diabetes, and how you can tell whether you are suffering from any of them. You need to know what you and your health care providers can do to prevent, detect, and treat diabetes-related psychological problems. Last but not least, we tell you about some promising new treatments for the condition.

Is there a quick way for you to check your psychological condition?

Everyone gets down in the dumps from time to time, even if they don't have diabetes. Having diabetes only makes it more likely that you will have some down times. If your blue periods are rare, pass quickly, and don't interfere much with your ability to take good care of yourself, you probably don't need the information in this chapter. If, on the other hand, emotional struggles are a regular part of your life with diabetes, read on.

What kind of psychological problems come with diabetes?

Diabetes-related psychological problems fall into two broad categories—coping difficulties and diagnosable psychological disorders. Coping difficulties are the more common problems, and diagnosable psychological disorders are the more serious ones. Let's talk about the serious ones first.

Some psychological problems to watch out for if you have diabetes are depression, anxiety disorder, and eating disorders. People with diabetes are more likely to have any of these problems, and these disorders tend to last longer, feel worse, and recur more often. In addition, having a psychological disorder makes diabetes management much more difficult.

What are the symptoms of depression?

Distinguishing between temporarily feeling blue and being truly depressed can be tricky, but we hope the signs and symptoms described below will help you decide which side of the line you are on.

Depression is probably the most common psychological disorder among people with diabetes. When most people say they are depressed, they don't use the term in the clinical sense. They are generally talking about feeling sad and dragged out emotionally in the way almost everyone does from time to time. These feelings come and go, usually in a couple of hours or a couple of days. Clinical depression is not like that; it takes you way down and keeps you there a long time. Clinical depression is diagnosed when a person has five or more specific symptoms for at least 2 weeks. Look at the symptoms in Table 16-1. If you have had at least five of the symptoms for at least that long, you may be suffering from clinical depression. A glance at this table makes it clear that depression really is different from a case of the blues.

Research strongly suggests that people with diabetes are more likely to suffer from clinical depression than are people who have no chronic medical condition. One study found that more than 40% of patients in an outpatient program at a large medical center reported symptoms indicating they could be clinically depressed. That's about three times the rate of depression in the general population.

If you studied Table 16-1 closely, you might notice something interesting: many of the symptoms listed there (specifically symptoms 2–6) look a lot like the symptoms

Table 16-1. Signs of Clinical Depression

1. Depressed mood (feeling sad or empty) most of the day nearly every day

2. Significant weight loss when not dieting, weight gain (for example, a change of more than 5% of body weight in a month), or decrease or increase in appetite nearly every day

3. Trouble sleeping or sleeping too much nearly every day

4. Feeling really agitated or physically sluggish nearly every day

5. Fatigue or loss of energy nearly every day

6. Markedly diminished interest or pleasure in all, or almost all, activities most of the day nearly every day

7. Feeling worthless or excessively or inappropriately guilty nearly every day

8. Diminished ability to think or concentrate, or indecisiveness, nearly every day

9. Recurrent thoughts of death (not just fear of dying), recurrent thoughts of suicide, a suicide attempt, or a specific plan to commit suicide

of hyperglycemia or high blood glucose. For this reason, it can sometimes be difficult to tell whether a person with diabetes who has these symptoms is depressed, hyperglycemic, or both. While it is important to sort this out, research indicates that when this overlap in symptoms is taken into account, depression is still more common among people with diabetes.

What puts you at risk for depression?

If depression is more common among people with diabetes, why is it so? Research has attempted to answer this question. First, there are some things that don't seem to explain the relationship—simply having diabetes didn't increase the risk of depression in the people studied, nor did the type of diabetes they had, how long they had diabetes, or the type of treatment they used to manage their diabetes. Even having a complication didn't increase the risk among the people studied. However, having several complications (three or more) did dramatically increase the risk of being depressed. That makes sense—at some point, the physical and emotional burden gets to be too much.

What is anxiety disorder?

Anxiety disorder is another serious psychological problem, found to be much more common among people who have diabetes than it is among the general population. Just as with depression, it's important to distinguish between normal anxiety and a diagnosable disorder. Everyone who has diabetes (in fact everyone who doesn't) worries about things sometimes. Some of these worries may be diabetes related; others may not be. Worrying about your blood sugars or about complications is normal, as is worrying about your job or your family.

A clinical anxiety disorder is different. When you have a clinical anxiety disorder, the worries are so intense, so uncomfortable, and so long lasting that they interfere with your ability to function at work, at home, and in other important areas of your life.

What are the symptoms of anxiety disorder?

You are probably suffering from a clinical anxiety disorder if you have been uncontrollably anxious for at least 6 months about a number of events or activities (such as work or school performance or your diabetes management) **and** during that period you had at least three of the symptoms listed in Table 16-2 for more days than you did not.

You probably noticed that some of these symptoms are identical to those of clinical depression. There is an overlap, because some psychological problems share similar

Table 16-2. Signs of Anxiety Disorder

1. Restlessness or feeling keyed up or on edge

2. Being easily fatigued

3. Difficulty concentrating or mind going blank

4. Irritability

5. Muscle tension

6. Sleep disturbance (difficulty falling or staying asleep, or restless, unsatisfying sleep)

symptoms, and because some people suffer from more than one disorder. This makes an important point: If you have any signs of a clinical psychological disorder, get help. You don't need to diagnose yourself to know that you need help.

What puts you at risk for anxiety disorder?

Clinical anxiety disorder is an exaggerated emotional reaction to fear, and people with diabetes can find a lot to fear, including hypoglycemia, complications, and the possible effects of diabetes on work and family life, to name just a few.

What are eating disorders?

Just as with depression and anxiety disorder, it is important to distinguish between normal behavior and behavior that indicates a problem. Spending a lot of time thinking about what you eat and carefully managing your eating are signs you are taking good care of your diabetes. Many people are concerned with eating and weight even if they don't have diabetes. Unfortunately, when these tendencies are combined, the result can be a full-blown eating disorder.

Eating disorders come in two forms. The first, which involves eating very, very little food often combined with extreme levels of exercise, is called *anorexia nervosa*. The other, which involves binge eating followed by purging, usually in the form of vomiting or the use of diuretics or laxatives, is called *bulimia nervosa*. It should come as no surprise that having either type of eating disorder enormously complicates diabetes care. In fact, there is no way you can effectively manage your diabetes if you have an active eating disorder.

What are the symptoms of an eating disorder?

How can you tell if your concern with eating and weight is normal? Many people want to be thin (and feel disappointed if they are not), exercise to manage weight and stay fit, and occasionally eat more than   they should. It is normal to eat prunes or use other approaches for occasional constipation and to use diuretics, when your doctor prescribes them, to treat fluid retention or high blood pressure. It is normal to adjust insulin doses to maintain good blood glucose control. It is not normal to engage in extreme forms of these behaviors. If you (or someone you care about) have any of the signs listed in Table 16-3, you may have an eating disorder.

What does insulin manipulation have to do with eating disorders?

Insulin manipulation is a frightening eating-disordered behavior unique to people with diabetes. This behavior is horrifyingly common. Some researchers estimate that as many as 50% of all young women frequently take less insulin than they need in an effort to control their weight. Decreasing the insulin leads to high blood glucose and loss of sugar (calories) and water in the urine. This causes weight loss but at a terrible price. Manipula-

Table 16-3. Signs of Eating Disorder

1. Weigh less than 85% of normal for your height, body frame, and age

2. Have an intense fear of gaining weight or becoming fat, even though you are underweight

3. See yourself as fat when others say you are too thin

4. Exercise far more than is necessary to stay fit

5. Miss at least three consecutive menstrual cycles

6. Deny the seriousness of your low body weight

7. Binge eat (eat very large amounts of food at a single sitting), at least twice a week for 3 months

8. Feel you can't stop eating or control what or how much you are eating

9. Vomit food you have eaten, or use diuretics, laxatives, enemas, or other medications to lose weight or prevent weight gain

10. Deliberately take less insulin than you need to maintain good blood glucose control with the conscious intent of managing your weight by passing some of the calories you consume as glucose in urine

tion of insulin doses to control or lose weight and other eating disorder behaviors can lead to acute emergencies and hospitalization and contribute to chronic complications.

What are the treatments for diabetes-related psychological disorders?

If you feel that you might be suffering from any of the psychological disorders just described, you should talk to your health care provider. First, tell your provider about your symptoms to be sure he or she knows what's going on. Then talk about treatment options. There are effective treatments for depression, anxiety disorder, and eating disorders. In our experience, the best treatment for these problems always involves counseling or psychotherapy and often involves medication as well.

We know that going into counseling can be a big step. Maybe you are a private person, and the idea of talking about your problems with someone you don't know might not sit right with you. You might not believe in psychotherapy. Naturally, you are the only one who can decide if counseling is for you, but you should seriously consider this option. Psychotherapy does work.

How can you find a counselor who fits your needs?

Unfortunately, counselors who specialize in treating people with diabetes are rare. If you can't find one, look for one who is willing to learn, through information you or your diabetes health provider can offer. You could also call the American Diabetes Association (ADA) at 1-800-342-2383 (1-800-DIABETES) or the American Association of Diabetes Educators (AADE) at 1-800-338-3633. They may be able to provide you with the name of a diabetes educator in your area who specializes in mental health services for people with diabetes.

Cognitive-behavioral therapy, which focuses on current problems and how to deal with them, is especially effective in treating diabetes-related psychological problems, so you might try to find a therapist who specializes in this approach.

What medicines are used to treat depression?

Medications can be a big help in treating depression and anxiety, but they are most effective when used in combination with counseling. Only a physician can tell whether medications would help you and prescribe the right one(s) for you. Here are some common ones.

Most antidepressants on the market today fall into one of two classes. The first class is *tricyclic antidepressants* and includes such drugs as Elavil (amitriptyline), Tofranil (imipramine), Sinequan (doxepin), and Pamelor (nortriptyline). Until recently, tricyclic antidepressants were by far the most commonly prescribed. That's less true today. Tricyclics may have side effects, including dry mouth, sleepiness, increased appetite and weight gain, and sexual dysfunction. Although most people don't experience these side effects, some of them can be especially troublesome for people with diabetes.

A newer class of antidepressants is *selective serotonin reuptake inhibitors* (SSRIs). Drugs in this class include Prozac (fluoxetine), Paxil (paroxetine), Zoloft (sertraline), Serzone (nefazodone), and Effexor (venlafaxine). These medications don't seem to make people as sleepy or contribute as much to sexual dysfunction. In addition, they actually tend to decrease appetite and lead to weight loss in some people. This is called a *benign side-effect profile*. It helps explain why so many prescriptions are being written for this class of antidepressants. SSRIs do cause gastrointestinal distress or overstimulation in some people.

If you start taking any antidepressant medication, it's important to keep in mind that the drug usually takes a couple of weeks or longer to begin producing its full beneficial effect. Unfortunately, the side effects begin much earlier (if you are going to experience any at all), and then they generally become less troublesome. So there may be a period of days or weeks after you begin taking an antidepressant when the only real effect you get will be a negative one. Be sure to tell the physician who prescribed the medication about both the benefits and side effects you are experiencing.

Are there medications for treating anxiety disorders?

If you are suffering from anxiety disorder, there are also medications that might help. Commonly prescribed anti-anxiety drugs include Ativan (lorazepam), BuSpar (buspirone), Serax (oxazepam), Tranxene (clorazepate), and Xanax (alprazolam).

Please keep in mind that the effectiveness of all mood-altering drugs is an individual matter. Different medications, even those closely related chemically, seem to affect different people differently. So you and your physician may need to try more than one medication before you find the right one for you.

Are there medications for treating eating disorders?

No medications are currently available that have been proven to be effective in treating eating disorders, though some researchers have reported success treating people with certain SSRI antidepressants.

What is the treatment for eating disorders?

For eating disorders, the most effective treatment is intensive psychotherapy. So, if you are suffering from an eating disorder, or if you suspect you might be, please get help. It is very difficult for people to admit they have an eating disorder.

We hear again and again from people how crucially important they feel it is to control their eating and how terrified they are at the prospect of giving up this control. Most people who suffer from eating disorders are terrified even to have anyone know about their problem because they feel deeply ashamed. You may believe no one can understand what you are going through or help you, but that's not true. Not everyone will understand or be able to help, but someone can. You need to find a mental health professional who treats people with eating disorders and hopefully knows something about diabetes as well.

What coping difficulties might you be likely to have?

As we mentioned earlier, diabetes overwhelmus takes two general forms. The more common form is coping diffi-culties. Just about everyone who has diabetes has had dif-ficulty coping from time to time. Often, these difficulties feel like mild forms of the psychological problems we've just talked about, especially depression and anxiety.

Although they aren't as serious as psychological disor-ders, coping problems make you uncomfortable and can get in the way of good diabetes self-care. Dealing with them is important. We focus on the more common day-to-day problems that you may face, such as dealing with discouragement, fear, whom to tell, what to eat, and how to find someone who knows what you're feeling.

If you're "demoralized," are you discouraged?

You don't need to have a psychological disorder like clini-cal depression to feel demoralized about living with dia-betes. Just the unending demands can be enough to do that. You are especially likely to feel demoralized when you experience one of the "crises" of diabetes. These crises include the original diagnosis of diabetes, failure of the treatment you are using (for example, oral medica-tions no longer work and you may have to start using insulin), or diagnosis of one of the complications of dia-betes (kidney, eye, or heart disease). When any of these events occur, you are likely to feel helpless, as though nothing you have done has been successful or that it is now too late to do anything about it.

It may help you to know that these reactions are com-mon. In fact, these events are referred to as "predictable crises" because so many people go through them. It's important to recognize that you can take action to dramatically reduce the impact of such events. A setback should not discourage you from continuing to fight the good fight. Some complications can be reversed, and others can be treated. Achieving or maintaining good glycemic control can prevent existing conditions from getting worse or the start of new ones. Most important, don't beat yourself up for anything that happened in the past. If you feel that you can do more to take better care of yourself, focus on what you can do now, not on what you did in the past. Some of the things you can do to get yourself back on track are discussed below.

What fears come with diabetes?

Fear is one of the most powerful emotions, even when it does not become so severe that it results in an anxiety disorder. Like anxiety, fear can be immobilizing. For example, fear of complications is one of the more common fears among people with diabetes. (Ironically, the fear can keep you from doing the things that would help prevent the complications!) Sometimes people use denial as a way of coping, but denying the possibility of complications will not make it go away. You have to find a way to acknowledge the fear and manage your disease.

Fear may also show up in other areas of diabetes management. Some people have a fear of sticking themselves to self-monitor blood glucose (SMBG) or to give themselves injections. Working closely with your health care provider, a diabetes educator, or a mental health professional familiar with diabetes can help you overcome fears like these.

If you take insulin, fear of hypoglycemia can keep you from trying for close-to-normal blood glucose levels.

Hypoglycemia is certainly nothing to be sneezed at. Severe hypoglycemia is always uncomfortable, it's often embarrassing, and it can even result in serious accidents if it occurs while you are driving or operating machinery. You may be tempted to allow your blood glucose to run higher than recommended to avoid these problems, but try not to give in to this temptation. Your doctor can help you revise your treatment to reduce the likelihood of hypoglycemia without sacrificing your health. You can take steps to avoid low blood glucose levels by checking more often and learning how your blood glucose is affected by things like exercise and stress, or times when insulin and food are out of synch. This process is called *blood glucose awareness training* and may be offered by a diabetes education program in your vicinity. Many diabetes education programs provide you with some help in dealing with fears about hypoglycemia.

You may also have fears about how diabetes will affect the rest of your life. You may fear that people will treat you differently because you have diabetes. Whom should you tell about your diabetes, and what should you tell them? While some people are very open in talking about their diabetes, most people are not and may wait until they know a person better before they open up. If you take insulin, there is more reason to let people know you have diabetes. Otherwise, they may misunderstand why you carry injection equipment, need to eat at certain times, and what is going on when you experience hypoglycemia.

Some parents have fears about their child with diabetes at school, and teachers may have fears, too. Education for parents, teachers, and classmates can help. One option is to obtain an excellent film for elementary school children called "The School Day and Diabetes

Basics for Teachers and Staff K-4." The film is available by writing to the Biomedical Communications Center for Educational Television, P.O. Box 19230, Southern Illinois University, Springfield, IL 62749.

Diabetes is not something to be ashamed about; it is a part of you. The closer you are to someone, the more important it is that they know about you. Even when you are in public, people are generally responsive if you tell them what you need, for example, "I need to get something to eat quickly because I have diabetes."

Finally, you may fear that having diabetes will affect your ability to get and hold a job. While a few careers are closed to people who have diabetes or those who take insulin, in most situations job-related discrimination based on the fact that you have diabetes is against the law. If you experience discrimination that you feel is illegal, you could contact a local ADA office. The ADA cannot give legal advice, but they may be able to advise you of existing remedies pertaining to your situation. In general, the Americans with Disabilities Act prevents people from discriminating against you because of your diabetes.

How does eating become a coping problem?

People eat to make themselves feel better. This can be unhealthy for anybody, but especially for people with diabetes. Although you may not engage in the binge/purge extremes of bulimia, you may find yourself overeating and feeling guilty about it, or not eating the number of vegetables and fruits that you know you need. Many people feel discouraged about their ability to eat as they should. This discouragement, along with the guilt, only makes matters worse, sapping the energy you need to get back on track. When you fall off the wagon (and everyone does), try to get right back on. One donut, or even several of them, is not going to ruin a diet unless you become discouraged and give up—and eat the rest of the donuts, too.

Being too controlled about what foods you eat is also a problem. Some people with diabetes become almost obsessed about food. They measure food portions and deny themselves even the smallest amount of "forbidden foods." Although it might work for some people for awhile, this type of behavior can lead to the bingeing pattern discussed above. If you deprive yourself of something that you really want, and then you do eat it, you may eat much more than you otherwise would, and feel guilty. You need to find an approach that you can live with over the long run rather than cycling back and forth between overcontrolled and undercontrolled eating.

What can you do for day-to-day diabetes problems?

If you are feeling overwhelmed by the demands of managing your diabetes, talk to your health care provider about ways to make your treatment plan less demanding. It might seem like wishful thinking but there's almost always a way to make diabetes self-care a little easier. It would probably help to join a diabetes support group and talk with people who know what you are going through. Discussing treatments with them may help you find other ways to make your diabetes management easier.

Another key to coping well with diabetes is the quality of your self-care. How well do you take care of yourself? It helps to stay current and master self-care skills. There are many sources of good information about the latest developments in diabetes research and treatment. ADA publishes two wonderful magazines called *Diabetes Forecast* and *Diabetes Advisor*, which you can get by joining ADA—call 1-800-806-7801. *Forecast* is like a *Time* or *Newsweek* and *Advisor* is like a *USA Today* or *Headline News* for people with diabetes. Information you find in any of these magazines can help you identify changes you might want to make in your diabetes self-care. Books on diabetes, available from ADA or in most large bookstores, are another excellent source of ideas. Then you can talk with your health care provider about new changes you are considering.

Where can you get help with learning and practicing self-care skills?

The fact is that information alone is not enough. You have to go beyond reading and hearing about useful treatments to learning how to do them. Think about one of your self-care skills that isn't as sharp as you'd like it to be. Now, how could you improve this skill? Would working with your health care provider help? Do you need a referral for help with your eating or exercise program, or glucose testing technique? You might even consider going to a diabetes education program where you can learn about all of the latest approaches to effective care. If you choose the last suggestion, be sure the program focuses on self-care *skills* and not on information alone. More and more insurance companies are realizing the value of diabetes education programs—they help you prevent serious complications and improve your day-to-day health—and your program may be covered by your health insurance.

Another source of help is diabetes counseling from a behavioral specialist (mental health counselor, psychologist, or social worker) or a behaviorally trained diabetes educator. These professionals can help you identify your personal barriers or "sticking points." We have found that being very specific is crucial to success in this process. The more specifically a sticking point is defined, the easier it is to solve. While some people might say that difficulty eating right is their sticking point; one man we know defined his problem more specifically, which made it a lot easier to work on. He said that he had an overpowering desire to snack between dinner and bedtime.

Once the specific sticking point is identified, the counselor can help you problem solve. Potential solutions are suggested, with emphasis on any approaches you have used successfully in the past. In the problem-solving process, you can learn to develop new perspectives that help you cope better with diabetes. Good problem-solving skills can be developed through practice, like any other skill. You can become your own diabetes counselor; in fact, there's no one in the world more qualified than you to do the job.

People with diabetes cope better when they get practical and emotional support from family and friends. If you think you are getting less support than you need, try to explain. Be calm, don't bring up the subject when you are upset. Talk about your needs, not how the other person failed you in the past. Accentuate the positive. Tell the person how he or she helped you in the past, and that what you are looking for is more of the same. If this approach doesn't work for you, consider making an appointment with your health care provider for yourself and your support person. You could ask the person to attend a diabetes support group meeting or a diabetes education class with you. These can all be good ways for you to help those who care about you be more helpful. It's easier for everyone to cope when they have a little help.

This chapter was written by Richard R. Rubin, PhD, CDE, and Mark Peyrot, PhD.

17

Men's Sexual Health

Case study

JG is a 32-year-old married man who came to his family practitioner with complaints of progressive loss of the ability to get and maintain an erection. He has had type 1 diabetes for 15 years and has good blood glucose control. In the past 3 years, he has developed some mild neuropathy in both his feet that comes and goes. Although he has maintained near-normal blood glucose levels in recent years, his previous history shows wide swings in glucose levels.

JG first noticed difficulty in maintaining an erection with some decrease in observed morning erections. Over the past 6 months, as neuropathy in his feet became more persistent, he noticed a decrease in the amount of ejaculate, but his feeling of orgasm continued. During the same time, his erectile function continued to decline, and, although he reports occasional partial morning erections, he has no erections satisfactory for sexual activity.

JG was referred to his urologist for evaluation and treatment of his erectile dysfunction and ejaculatory changes.

Introduction

Male erectile dysfunction, or impotence, may be defined as an inability to have and maintain an erection rigid enough for sexual intercourse. It has been estimated that more than 18 million American men suffer from erectile dysfunction. It is three times more common in men with diabetes in any age-group. The Massachusetts Male Aging Study (MMAS), the first large-scale study on sexual dysfunction of a general population, evaluated 1,709 randomly chosen men from the Boston suburbs. Of these men, 1,290 (75.5%) completed questionnaires concerning their sexual function. It may surprise you that more than half (52%) of these healthy middle-aged men complained of erectile dysfunction. The study showed that the likelihood of any man having erectile dysfunction increases with age.

The MMAS also reviewed impotence in middle-aged men with diabetes. This and other studies show that diabetes in men more than 40 years old is associated with increasing erectile dysfunction. In this group as a whole, impotence was 11% more common than in the non-diabetic group.

Nonetheless, there is hope. There are ways to diminish your risks and to improve your overall health, which will improve your libido (interest in sex) and enjoyment.

Are there ways of predicting who will have erectile dysfunction?

In the MMAS, the factors that researchers found helpful in predicingt who would have some degree of impotence included alcohol intake, level of blood glucose control, and whether the man had intermittent claudication (pain in the legs while walking, a sign of vascular disease in the legs), retinopathy, or neuropathy (nerve damage).

What puts you at risk for developing impotence?

Impotence can be caused by physical conditions, injury, or emotional or psychological conditions or as a side effect of medications that you are taking. It can be caused by drugs such as alcohol or marijuana.

Medical problems associated with impotence include heart disease, hypertension, and high cholesterol (hyperlipidemia). This is no surprise, because all of these abnormalities relate to circulation. And your risk of developing circulation problems is intensified by cigarette smoking. Having poor blood glucose control for long periods of time also puts you at risk for developing impotence. JG had wide swings in blood glucose levels for several years and was suffering from peripheral neuropathy in his feet as a result. His problems achieving an erection could be due to nerve damage, which can result from poor glucose control.

Psychological risk factors associated with impotence (both in men with diabetes and in otherwise healthy individuals) include depression, anger, and low self-esteem. These are as powerful as any physical factor and often contribute to the problem even if they are not the main cause. JG is a young man and is having emotional difficulty accepting his loss of sexual function.

The drugs you take for other conditions can also put you at risk for impotence. These drugs include blood pressure drugs such as beta blockers and diuretics, some antidepressants, and some stomach ulcer medications. Over-the-counter medications can also cause problems, as can recreational drugs such as alcohol and marijuana. Discuss with your health care provider whether any medication that you are taking is causing or adding to your experience of impotence (Table 17-1).

On rare occasions, low levels of testosterone will put you at risk for impotence.

How does an erection normally occur?

The complex process that results in an erection includes emotions, hormones, blood circulation, and nerves. Nerve pathways to and from the brain can initiate (or

Table 17-1. Medications Associated with Male Erectile Dysfunction

Anti-Hypertensive (High blood pressure)	1. Diuretics 2. Vasodilators 3. Central sympatholytics 4. Ganglion blockers 5. Beta blockers 6. ACE inhibitors 7. Calcium-channel blockers
Antiandrogens (testosterone)	1. Estrogens 2. Luteinizing-hormone–releasing hormone agonists
Anticholinergics	1. Atropine 2. Propantheline 3. Diphydramine
Antidepressants	1. Tricyclines 2. Monoamine oxidase inhibitors 3. Serotonin re-uptake inhibitors
Antianxiety Drugs	1. Benzodiazepines 2. Phenothiazines 3. Butyrophenones
Miscellaneous	1. Alcohol 2. Marijuana 3. Cocaine 4. Barbiturates 5. Nicotine 6. Cimetidine 7. Clofibrate 8. Digoxin 9. Indomethacin

inhibit) your erectile response. Seeing or imagining things that are sexually exciting and touching or having your penis touched activate these signals from the brain. There are changes in blood circulation that allow more blood to flow into and be "dammed up" in the penis. This forms the rigid structure of an erection. Both the inflow and the damming of the blood are necessary for the erection to occur and be maintained. This is all done under the influence of nerves that work automatically,— the autonomic nerves.

What part do hormones play in the erection process?

Male hormone, or testosterone, is essential for erectile function. Also, hormones in the central nervous system influence sexual activity by increasing libido and sexual behavior. If you are less and less interested in sex, you might have low male hormone levels, but this condition is relatively uncommon. If you do need testosterone replacement, your health care provider can determine why it is low and can give you testosterone in one of several forms.

What can cause erectile dysfunction in a man with diabetes?

There can be many causes. It may be a result of peripheral neuropathy (nerve damage), atherosclerosis (clogged arteries), or decreased testosterone levels. Impotence can be caused by prescription medications for high blood pressure, such as beta blockers and diuretics, for depression, for ulcers, or to prevent vomiting. It can be caused or made worse by psychological factors. It can be caused by injury. The most common physical causes of impotence with diabetes are blood vessel disease with decreased circulation and nerve damage. Both of these conditions are complications of diabetes. Add to these health problems the stress of worries and fears about aging, diabetes, complications, and sexual performance and you have the formula for erectile dysfunction.

What is ejaculatory dysfunction?

Peripheral neuropathy appears to be responsible for the ejaculatory abnormalities frequently encountered in as many as 32% of men with diabetes. The most common of these dysfunctions is the one JG encountered, a decrease in the amount of ejaculate (retrograde ejaculation). Retrograde ejaculation is ejaculation backward into the   bladder. It is caused by nerve dysfunction and can occasionally be overcome by the use of certain drugs. If you suspect that this is your problem, you should consult a urologist or your primary health care provider.

How is erectile dysfunction diagnosed?

JG's appointment with his health care provider began with a full history, complete physical examination, and appropriate laboratory tests. Sometimes, male erectile dysfunction may be the first indication of diabetes or vascular disease.

JG's initial history included the date when his erectile dysfunction began (6 months earlier) and the presence or absence of previous erectile function (it had never happened before). JG's provider asked whether his erectile dysfunction was accompanied by ejaculatory dysfunction, diminished interest in sex, or failure to reach orgasm. To determine the possible causes, your provider needs to know about the last episode of successful sexual intercourse, how often erectile problems occur, whether you have nighttime and morning erections or erections during masturbation, and whether you have erectile dysfunction only with a certain partner or situation.

How are psychological causes of impotence diagnosed?

Men with psychological impotence will still have morning, nighttime, and self-stimulated erections. The onset of erectile dysfunction in these men is often sudden and may be related to a specific life event. If this is the case, your provider would take a more detailed psychosexual history exploring the sources of anxiety, relationship problems, stress, and possible depression.

Erectile dysfunction from physical causes is more often a gradual loss of rigidity with decreases in morning and nighttime erections, much like JG's experience.

What other questions will your health care provider ask?

Your provider will ask about any medications you are taking. Sexual dysfunction is frequently caused by high blood pressure medications such as diuretics and vasodilators. Antidepressant medications may allow you to maintain an erection but may make ejaculation more difficult. The other drugs that can influence erections and ejaculation are listed in Table 17-1. Your provider will ask whether you drink alcohol or smoke and how often.

What happens during your physical examination?

Your physical examination should include the external genitalia, prostate, lower-extremity pulses, and hair distribution on the feet and legs. You'll also have your blood pressure, cardiac status, and lower-extremity pulses checked to see whether circulation problems are contributing to sexual dysfunction.

What laboratory tests need to be done?

Laboratory tests must include a urine analysis and blood glucose level. Elevated blood glucose in a patient with erectile dysfunction are sometimes how his diabetes is first diagnosed. Blood levels of testosterone and other hormone studies may be important in identifying specific causes for organic (physical) erectile dysfunction.

How is male erectile dysfunction treated?

Impotence can be treated in several ways, depending on whether it is brought on by physical or emotional causes. There are both oral and injection drugs, physical devices, and surgical implants. You and your health care provider will choose a treatment based on the physical and psychological factors affecting your condition.

What if your testosterone levels are too low?

It is unusual that you would need testosterone replacement. However, if your blood tests indicate it, there are a couple of ways this can be done—by injection or transdermal skin patches. Oral tablets are seldom used because they do not work as well as the patch and may be toxic to your liver.

Normal testosterone concentrations vary throughout the day, with the highest levels appearing early in the morning and the lowest around midnight. Testosterone injected into the muscles fails to reproduce this diurnal variation in testosterone concentration and produces a very high initial concentration of testosterone that falls to a level below normal before the next injection. So a transdermal patch was developed.

Testosterone skin patches have been available for the past several years. These can be applied over muscles or on the scrotum for testosterone replacement. The treatment requires daily application of testosterone patches, which produces serum testosterone levels similar to normal levels. Patients report improvement in energy level, mood, strength, libido and sexual function, and in nighttime erections while on testosterone patches. The patch can cause skin irritation and itching, but these side effects are usually temporary and can be treated with topical agents.

Are there pills for impotence?

Yohimbine, an oral medication for erectile dysfunction, comes from the bark of the pausinystalin yohimbe tree and has been used for more than a century as an aphrodisiac (a substance thought to enhance sexual desire). Studies in men with psychologically caused impotence have demonstrated a positive response in 31% of men taking yohimbine. There have been no clinical trials of this drug only in men with diabetes, mainly because men with diabetes do not complain of impotence until it is beyond the stage where yohimbine will help. Yohimbine tends to help patients who still have erections but have a rigidity problem; most patients with diabetes have lost both when they come for treatment. Penile rings seem to work almost as well, if not better, than yohimbine for this problem or can be used in combination with it. You can use a penis ring with the medicated urethral system for erection (MUSE, discussed below) as well, if you achieve better results that way.

New drugs are or will soon be available to stimulate erectile function. Apomorphine is a pill you place under your tongue, and it stimulates central nervous system control of erectile function. One of the most talked about new agents is sildenafil (Viagra), which stimulates and maintains erectile function. Its affect appears to be most significant when taken 30–60 minutes before intercourse. Although studies specific to diabetic men have not been performed for either apomorphine or sildenafil, these agents work well on a wide variety of causes of male erectile dysfunction.

What about injection treatments for erectile dysfunction?

During the early 1980s, medications were found that could create erections in impotent men when injected into the penis. A variety of drugs are available, have been used throughout the world, and have rehabilitated many diabetic men with chronic impotence. Unless you have severe vascular disease, injection therapy appears to be one of the most effective methods for restoring potency.

What do you need to learn about using these drugs?

The first time you use an injectable drug should be in an erectile dysfunction clinic to learn the proper technique and to monitor the effectiveness of the drug and any side effects, such as prolonged erections. The first dose is low, to demonstrate the injection technique. Doses are increased until you get a good-quality erection that does not last too long.

Then, you will be shown how to fill the syringe. An area at the side of the penis is chosen, and the skin is cleansed with alcohol. Then, the skin is held tight, and the needle is placed in the corporus cavernosum (erectile tissue) at the base of the penis. This can be performed on either side, avoiding superficial veins. If the erection is inadequate, an increased dose is used with the next demonstration, 24–48 hours later.

What are the side effects of self-injection therapy?

Side effects of self-injection therapy include treatment failure, an increase in thickened tissue, prolonged erection, and penile pain. A prolonged erection may require the use of aspiration and irrigation techniques.

Are there other treatments for impotence don't use injections?

There is a method called the *medicated urethral system for erection* (MUSE). Alprostadil (prostaglandin E_1) is a tiny suppository that is inserted virtually painlessly with an applicator into the opening at the end of the penis. This system works much like injection therapy but without a needle and is effective for most users. Or you may want to try sildenafil (Viagra), an oral medication you take 30–60 minutes before intercourse. It has been shown to be effective for a large majority of users.

What are the side effects of these other systems?

Side effects of the MUSE system include low blood pressure in a few patients and penile pain in as many as one-third of patients. Viagra does not seem to interact with the medications you might be taking such as ACE inhibitors or antidepressants. A few users report headaches, flushing, or vision changes such as a color tinge or fuzziness.

What are vacuum constriction devices?

The vacuum device consists of a long, clear plastic tube (vacuum chamber), pump, and constriction band, which is applied to the base of the penis after erection is achieved. The vacuum chamber is attached to a vacuum pump on one end and open on the other. This open end is placed over the penis, and a seal is obtained at the base with lubricant jelly. The pump mechanism creates a vacuum of approximately 100 mmHg, pulling blood into the penis and creating an erection. Once the erection has become complete, an elastic ring is moved from the tube around the base of the penis to prevent blood from flowing back out of the penis. These devices are used widely by patients with diabetes or vascular disease or after radical surgery. Satisfaction achieved is about the same as from an erection achieved by other methods.

Are there any side effects from use of the vacuum device?

Side effects from the vacuum constriction device include feeling cold and numb during erection, with difficulty ejaculating because of the ring. Some patients have difficulty obtaining orgasm as a result of this feeling. Changes in penile skin as well as penile curvature have been reported from frequent use of the vacuum erection device. The ring can cause tissue damage. Despite these problems, patient and partner satisfaction appeared to be satisfactory in many studies.

Are penile rings used alone?

A penile ring is an elastic band that is placed at the base of the erect penis to keep blood in it (maintaining the erection) during intercourse. Rings may be used alone or in combination with the vacuum device, injections, or MUSE system.

Is vascular surgery a treatment for impotence?

Vascular bypass surgery is appropriate only for select younger patients without generalized vascular abnormalities who have erectile dysfunction caused by injury to the external genitals or the arteries in the penis. Procedures used for this group of patients are generally not appropriate for patients with erectile dysfunction caused by diabetes.

What about surgical implants or penile prostheses?

Before there was widespread use of drug therapies for erectile dysfunction, more than 50% of patients undergoing implantation of penile prostheses had diabetes. This therapy is not popular now and is generally chosen by men who are not satisfied with the results they get from other methods. The many models of penile prostheses available can be divided into inflatable and semirigid types. All implants provide rigidity and size to the penile shaft and are enough like a normal erection to permit intercourse. The degree of flaccidity (how soft they become) between uses, however, varies with the type of device. The prosthetic devices are usable within 4–6 weeks of surgical implantation.

The inflatable penile prosthesis is available in a self-contained, two-piece, or three-piece design. The three-piece design appears the most normal, providing the best possible erection. Self-contained penile prostheses are combinations of the semirigid rod and inflatable prostheses and contain a pump at the tip end of the penis on each cylinder and a reservoir at the base. Once surgically implanted, the prosthesis is inflated by pressing on the pump and deflated by deflecting the penis actively to activate the release valve. These cylinders have limited inflatable portions and cannot be expanded or deflated very much. They may still be somewhat rigid between uses.

What are the side effects of surgical penile implants?

The most difficult complication is that of infection, which occurs in approximately 3% of patients with penile prostheses. Higher infection rates have been reported in patients with autoimmune diseases, transplants, and diabetes. Other complications include breaking or leaking of the fluid in the prosthesis, sustained pain, reduced penile

length, and reduced sensation. These are rare but significant enough to concern you, your partner, and your surgeon.

Is there a way to prevent impotence?

The most important step you can take to prevent impotence is to avoid the one-two punch of poor circulation
and nerve damage—that is, to maintain good blood glucose control, good blood pressure control, and good cholesterol levels. Many studies have shown that nerve
function is preserved in patients who have near-normal
blood glucose levels. There is also strong evidence that
good blood glucose control delays the development of
vascular disease. Stop smoking. Exercise. Ask your doctor
about the side effects of any medications that you have to
take.

In conclusion

Male erectile dysfunction is a common complication of
diabetes. It is usually caused by peripheral neuropathy,
cardiovascular disease, psychological problems, or combinations of the three. If you have erectile dysfunction, it is
important to consult with an expert for careful diagnosis
and appropriate treatment.

Culley C. Carson, MD, contributed to this chapter.

18

Women's Sexual Health

Case study

LO, a 46-year-old woman diagnosed with type 2 diabetes 5 years ago, has always maintained good glucose control. She and her husband have been married 20 years and have three children. Through most of their marriage, they have enjoyed an active sex life. Lately, however, LO no longer initiates sex and finds ways to avoid it. Even when she feels emotionally aroused, she takes a long time to feel physically aroused and then experiences discomfort during intercourse. As a first step, the doctor suggests an over-the-counter vaginal lubricant and that she talk to her husband about what she has been experiencing.

Case study

Mrs. B, a 36-year-old with type 1 diabetes for 27 years, came to her physician to plan a pregnancy. She had high blood pressure and protein in her urine. She had high blood glucose levels and a glycated hemoglobin level of 9.8% (normal range is up to 6). Her insulin therapy consisted of two insulin injections a day.

Mrs. B's blood pressure needed to come down before she got pregnant and the protein in her urine was too high. Her physician was also concerned about retinopathy. She was referred to an ophthalmologist for laser therapy to new blood vessels at the edge of her retina. Her retinas were then in good shape for the pregnancy. A nephrologist placed Mrs. B on blood pressure lowering drugs considered safe for pregnancy. Her health care team helped her with a program of diet, exercise, and medication to bring her blood glucose levels close to normal with 3 or 4 insulin injections a day (intensive insulin therapy) and blood glucose monitoring 6 to 8 times a day.

After 6 months, her glycated hemoglobin was in the normal range, and her blood pressure was less than 130/80 mmHg. Mrs. B was given the "go-ahead" to become pregnant. During the pregnancy, her blood pressure, blood glucose levels, and health status all remained unchanged. She delivered a healthy, 7-pound baby boy.

Introduction

Some women define sexuality as the ability to bear children. This definition tends to devalue the whole woman. It ignores how important it is to feel fulfilled by the intimacy, pleasure, and satisfaction of two people connecting with each other. Sexuality is as important to a woman in her 60s as it is to a woman in her 30s. Women with diabetes can have a healthy and sexually fulfilling life.

What sexual problems can happen to any woman?

It may help to divide sexual problems into two categories: sexual difficulties and sexual dysfunction.

Sexual difficulties

Sexual difficulties are problems in the relationship and communication between two people that impact their sexual activity. Generally, these difficulties are a result of lack of knowledge of each other's sexual needs and preferences. They do not or cannot tell each other what they want. A woman will complain that her partner wants sex too often or not often enough, that he does not engage in enough foreplay, or that there is no affectionate closeness after intercourse. She may feel unattracted to her partner, dislike his habits or sexual practices, or be unable to relax with him in sexual play.

Sexual dysfunctions

Sexual dysfunctions are problems with the physical processes. Human sexual response normally consists of four events in sequence: desire, arousal, orgasm, and satisfaction. Different physiological processes are involved in each phase, so you may have difficulty in one phase but not the others.

Desire is defined for both sexes as the motivation or wish to have a sexual experience. It frequently is a response to an external cue such as an erotic picture or genital pressure. This is an activity that begins in the brain and depends on a certain blood level of hormones. Degree of desire, however, is not dependent on levels of hormones.

Arousal is the emotional and physiological response to mental or tactile erotic stimulation and is expressed both as a feeling of excitement and as genital vasocongestion (accumulation of blood), the primary physiological measure of sexual response. It is demonstrated by vaginal lubrication.

Orgasm, primarily orchestrated by the nervous system, is characterized by a series of rhythmic contractions of the muscles of the internal reproductive structures and vagina. Some women may have several consecutive orgasms before experiencing relaxation and pleasure, and some may be unable to reach orgasm at all.

Dyspareunia is genital pain that occurs during or after intercourse when there is inadequate lubrication. *Vaginismus* is the involuntary contraction of the vaginal muscles that interferes with vaginal penetration by the penis or sometimes even fingers.

The most common problem that women report is low sexual desire—30–50% of women seeing sex or marital therapists complain of desire problems.

What causes sexual dysfunctions?

Sexual dysfunctions can be caused by any disease or medication that interferes with the hormones, brain and nerve involvement, blood circulation, or muscular portions of sexual response. Additionally, pain or disability can interfere. Just as important are psychological factors. Several physical and emotional factors can interact to produce sexual dysfunctions and sexual difficulties in women.

What are the symptoms of sexual problems in women with diabetes?

Some women with type 1 diabetes have difficulty becoming physically aroused. They may have less vaginal thickening and lubrication. Both penile erection and vaginal lubrication depend on the increase of blood flow to the genital area. Along with vaginal dryness, an inadequate accumulation of blood in the genital area can cause irritation or pain with sexual activity.

Type 2 diabetes, on the other hand, puts a woman at significant risk for developing difficulties with her sexual relationships and sexual dysfunctions. Older women with type 2 diabetes may have more sexual problems than their age-group, including low sexual desire, poor vaginal lubrication, painful intercourse, difficulty reaching orgasm by any method, and less satisfaction. More of these women report that they use lubricants. Even though their actual frequency of intercourse and masturbation does not differ from women without diabetes, women with type 2 have reported being much less satisfied with almost every aspect of their sexual relationship. Fear of rejection or the negative consequences of future complications affect many women.

What puts you at risk for developing sexual problems?

The damage that the high levels of blood glucose in diabetes can do to your blood vessels and nerves affects both circulation and sensation. Clearly, this damage may affect what you can feel and how you respond.

Persistent high blood glucose levels can increase your chance of vaginitis (inflammation of the vagina) or yeast infections. If you have problems with unusual discharge from the vagina, itching, or yeast infections, you should consult with your doctor to determine the best treatment for correcting the problem and improving your blood glucose control. High blood glucose can also sap your energy and sense of vitality. Feeling sluggish and tired can interfere with how attracted and receptive you are to engaging in sexual activity.

Being able to enjoy the wide range of physical and emotional feelings associated with sexual contact is linked to your emotional state. This can have as powerful an effect on sexual dysfunction as a physical problem.

Women who have multiple health problems may be taking medications that interfere with their ability to have fulfilling sexual contact. Some medications can interfere with your desire to have sex (libido). Others cause drying of the vaginal tissue, which leads to painful intercourse. Ask your doctor about the effects of your medications on your sexual health.

How does diabetes affect the sexual functioning of older women?

As menopause approaches and the vagina loses a degree of elasticity and lubrication, the effects of diabetes may become more apparent. The diminished circulation to the vaginal area that diabetes can cause leads to poor nerve responses, or even depletes some of the neurotransmitters in the genital tissue. Pain and difficulty reaching orgasm are the result.

Women who develop type 2 diabetes generally do so in middle age, well after their sex roles and marital patterns are established. It is possible that the intrusion of the disease and its restricted regimen at this time in her life may undermine a woman's self-image, cause major readjustments in lifestyle, and produce or aggravate marital tensions. In fact, women with type 2 diabetes have reported that the disease has a damaging effect on relationships and produces more family problems. Emotionally, they experience more mood swings and anxiety than before the disease developed and feel more inadequate and less flexible. The onset of diabetes can signal the end of one's sexual attractiveness and desirability and raise concerns about earlier aging. For example, because women with type 2 are more likely to be overweight, it is possible that discomfort with their own body images and their partners' reactions may inhibit their sexual relationships.

Should you be concerned about your diabetes during sex?

If you take insulin or oral hypoglycemic medication, you may be concerned that the physical exertion of sex will result in low blood glucose. You could consider reducing the appropriate amount of insulin before having sex, or you can choose to eat something before having sex. If low blood glucose does occur, you may find that you are unable to perform as usual and cannot enjoy the experience. It will be important to discuss with your partner the potential for low blood glucose, the symptoms, and the treatment.

Does diabetes affect your monthly cycles?

If you are still menstruating, you may have noticed your blood glucose values are higher around or during your period. Blood glucose is affected by the natural release of hormones that cause your body to be more resistant to its own insulin or to insulin that you inject. Normally, blood glucose remains high for 3–5 days and gradually returns to the level it was before your period.

During PMS, menstruation, or menopause, you might have less energy and not want to exercise. If you stop exercising, your blood glucose may rise even higher. Your ability to control food cravings and to continue with your exercise program will help you balance your blood glucose. Chart your responses during your cycle. Also note the effect of caffeine and alcohol on blood glucose levels at these times. Women with uncontrolled blood glucose may have irregular monthly cycles and acne.

What do your provider and diabetes educator need to know?

Female patients, especially older ones, are often reluctant to raise the subject of sexuality with their providers, believing that their concerns are embarrassing, trivial, or inappropriate unless the provider brings up the topic. It may not be easy to communicate your concerns to your partner or to your provider. Yet, if you want to honor yourself as a woman and this is an issue for you, take the risk. You need to let your provider know if you have noticed any changes in your sex life that could be related to your diabetes. Do you have

- a decrease in sexual desire or interest?
- vaginal dryness or tightness with intercourse?
- pain or discomfort with intercourse?
- pain at penetration or with deep thrusting?
- soreness and irritation after sexual activity?
- more difficulty reaching an orgasm than in the past?
- less satisfaction with your sexual relationship now than previously?

To assess the possible emotional causes of your sexual dysfunction, your provider needs to know the following:

1. What was your level of sexual activity and responsiveness (frequency, variation, initiation) before diabetes?
2. What are the sexual needs and expectations of you and your partner?
3. What other or underlying difficulties are the two of you having?
4. How do you feel about having diabetes? To what extent does it interfere with your life and relationship?
5. What effect do you feel diabetes has had on your relationship in general and your sexual relationship in particular?

Why is it helpful to know when the problem began?

It helps to know when the sexual problem began to determine what may be the cause and whether it is related to diabetes complications or psychosocial adjustment. It is also helpful to know whether the problem is generalized (occurs in every sexual situation or with different partners) or situational (occurs only during specific sexual activities).

Does your spouse or partner need to speak with your provider?

Of course. Your spouse or sexual partner plays an important role in treatment or counseling. Your partner's viewpoint on any sexual problems or any changes in your sexual relationship that may be attributed to the diabetes might help you find and treat the cause—and improve communication between you. Chronic illness can place stress and strain even on strong relationships. It is important to assess how your partner is affected by the illness, because this can impact your sexual relationship, too.

It is also important to know whether concerns about pregnancy are affecting a couple's sex life. Infertility treatment often temporarily disrupts sexual pleasure. On the other hand, fear of pregnancy can interfere with sexual desire and activity.

What can you expect from treatment?

If your sexual problem is mild, began recently, or has a strong diabetes-related cause, some practical and brief interventions by your health care team may be effective.

If your sexual problems are long standing or complicated, you probably need to work with both your physician for treatment of your diabetes and a counselor or therapist in sexual, marital, or individual counseling. You may need accurate sexual education about normal sexual behaviors—there are many excellent books on the subject. It helps many women to realize that their concerns, thoughts, fantasies, and experiences are normal and shared by many other women.

What part do hormones play in the treatment of sexual dysfunction?

A woman who has lost ovarian function or is post-menopausal may experience less desire for sex because of a hormonal deficiency. Estrogen replacement can improve vaginal elasticity and lubrication, but additional supplementation with male sex hormones (androgens) is more likely to directly increase sexual desire. Although androgen therapy has been helpful to women who undergo surgical menopause, it has no documented benefit for premenopausal women with low sexual desire.

The arousal-phase problem of poor vaginal lubrication is often easy to treat. A woman who has low estrogen levels can use replacement estrogen as a pill, patch, or vaginal cream. The estrogen can actually reverse vaginal atrophy within a few months. For premenopausal diabetic women or for those postmenopausal patients who have risk factors preventing estrogen replacement, vaginal lubricants are quite helpful.

Are there exercises you can do as part of the treatment for sexual difficulties?

To minimize pain during intercourse, you can learn to relax the pubococcygeal muscles. You can identify these muscles by contracting them during urination and noticing that the flow stops. You can put a finger inside of the vagina before squeezing the muscles and feel the slight vaginal contraction. Once you have found the muscles, you can practice squeezing them for a count of 3 and then releasing them, 10 times in a row. If vaginal penetration for intercourse feels tight and painful, you can tense and relax the muscles before and during the process. Patients who have pain on penetration or with deep thrusting should use positions that give you more control. These include sitting or kneeling over your partner or both partners lying on your sides facing each other.

Is difficulty in reaching orgasm a separate problem in women with diabetes?

No. Rather, it is often a product of lessened desire and arousal or physical discomfort during sex. Before assuming the trouble is related to neuropathy, your physician may ask if you are orgasmic with clitoral stimulation (by your hand, with a vibrator, or from a partner). Many healthy women have a difficult time reaching orgasm from penile-vaginal thrusting alone, and the woman with orgasmic difficulty may simply require more adequate clitoral stimulation to reach orgasm.

When might you be referred to a specialist?

A referral to a specialist in sexual problems is indicated under the following conditions:

- The sexual problem is severe or has been present for several years.
- The problem does not respond to primary care team intervention.
- The patient is poorly adjusted psychologically or has a highly conflicted close relationship.
- The problem does not appear to be related to diabetes.

For most women's sexual problems, the referral of choice is to a mental health professional who has special training in treating sexual dysfunctions. The most common causes of sexual problems in women with diabetes are psychological—depression, anxiety about attractiveness, poor sexual communication, relationship conflict, or a history of a traumatic sexual experience. A competent specialist is likely to be a fully qualified social worker, psychiatrist, or psychologist who has specialty training at the postgraduate level. These professionals can often be located on the faculty of a local psychology department or medical school. County or state mental health organizations can also provide referrals. Professional organizations, such as the Society for Sex Therapy and Research, are also sources of reliable referrals.

How do you know if depression is related to your sexual difficulties?

Loss of desire for sex is often related to depression. If you also have disturbed sleep, a change in appetite for food, depressed mood, chronic fatigue, physical symptoms without clear cause, and trouble with concentration or memory, you probably could benefit from treatment for depression. Antidepressant drugs and brief symptom-focused psychotherapy are both effective. Also, any problem with the couple that decreases communication or increases anger may negatively impact on sexual desire.

When might you be referred to a gynecologist?

A gynecologist is especially helpful with dysfunctions related to menopause or to genital pain. The examination should assess tenderness around the vagina, the condition of Bartholin's glands (which secrete vaginal lubrication), the mucous membranes of the vagina, and the presence of pain deep in the vagina or pelvis with pressure or movement of the cervix and uterus. Women who have vulvar (external genitalia) tenderness, burning, and pain with sexual stimulation sometimes have a syndrome known as *vulvar vestibulitis.* Inflammation of numerous glands around the vaginal opening can be diagnosed with colposcopy. Common causes of pain only on deep thrusting include endometriosis, pelvic adhesions, abnormalities of the uterine ligaments, or ovarian cysts. However, none of these gynecological problems has been associated with diabetes.

Does diabetes cause any problems when choosing contraception?

Decisions about the best contraceptive methods should be made with your partner and your physician. Options range from abstinence to the pill. In the past, a woman with diabetes was advised against taking the pill for two reasons. First, taking oral contraceptives could worsen her blood glucose control. Even today, a woman may find that this is true. Second, she may be at risk of developing problems with circulation and clotting, such as heart attack or stroke. Because the dose of estrogen and progestin has been decreased in newer pills, so has the risk for these problems.

Women on the pill who smoke are at greater risk for circulation problems. Smoking causes the blood vessels to narrow, the walls of the vessels to thicken, and the blood to clot. That's why it is important for a woman to quit smoking. High glycated hemoglobin (HbA_{1c}) levels (indicating poor blood glucose control) or being dehydrated may also increase your chances of having blood clotting problems.

A new oral medication for type 2 diabetes, troglitazone (Rezulin), can decrease the effectiveness of estrogen by 30%. If you take troglitazone while you are on a low-dose birth control pill, you may have breakthrough bleeding (bleeding between periods) or may even become pregnant. If you are on the pill and taking troglitazone, ask your physician if your birth control pill needs to be changed. Also, use a backup method of birth control the first couple of months that you are taking troglitazone.

It is important for a woman on the pill to have her blood fats and blood pressure checked regularly. If you have high blood pressure or high blood fats, you may need to use a different method of contraception. Taking the pill when you have high blood pressure can increase the chance that eye or kidney disease will get worse. The pill can also cause a rise in blood fat levels (cholesterol, LDL, and triglyceride levels). Barrier methods, such as the diaphragm or condoms, have no effect on blood glucose or blood fats. Speak with your provider about the best options for you.

How does diabetes affect pregnancy?

Women with diabetes need to establish near-normal blood glucose levels **before** getting pregnant, because the baby's organs (heart, brain, lungs, and kidneys, etc.) are formed in the first 8 weeks of pregnancy, almost before the woman knows she is pregnant. Also, your own well-being during pregnancy depends on your health before you become pregnant. If you maintain normal blood glucose and see your health care team regularly, you and the child should be fine. If you already have complications, especially retinopathy or nephropathy, they may get worse. You, your spouse, and your physician have to weigh the benefits against the risks before you get pregnant.

If you take a sulfonylurea, you cannot take it during pregnancy. Even if you do not use insulin, you may need it during pregnancy. And you may need to check your blood glucose more often (6 to 8 times a day).

Women who develop diabetes only during pregnancy, called *gestational diabetes,* do not have the same risks as a woman with diabetes before she gets pregnant. You don't have complications of diabetes, and your baby's organs are formed before the diabetes develops. To keep the baby from being too large (macrosomic) in response to your high blood glucose levels, you should also follow a meal plan, and you may need insulin to keep your blood glucose levels normal. A large child may need to be delivered by cesarean section (C-section).

Realize that as soon as you deliver the baby, your insulin needs return to your normal level. If you breast-feed, you may have low blood sugars that are more severe and occur more often than before you were pregnant. See a dietitian before and during pregnancy to be sure you're getting the calories you need. Snacking is important to cover bedtime and middle-of-the-night feedings.

How might your diabetes affect your baby?

If you have near-normal blood glucose levels throughout pregnancy, from conception through delivery, your child has the same low risk of birth defects as any other child. The infant of a mother with diabetes usually weighs more than normal, which can lead to birth injuries, such as a broken clavicle (collarbone). If your blood glucose is high during labor, your baby may have hypoglycemia once the umbilical cord is cut. Low blood glucose sets in 1 to 3 hours after birth and should be checked during the first two days of life. Although the baby may be large, its lungs may not be mature, and sometimes, breathing difficulties occur. If you have type 1 diabetes, your child is a little more likely to develop diabetes (1–4%). If you have type 2, your child's risk is 1 in 7. Your child is more likely to be obese after puberty, so give him or her a healthy lifestyle of well-balanced meals and plenty of exercise.

How are menopause and diabetes connected?

Each woman experiences menopause differently. Your experience will be influenced by your body, your attitudes and fears about menopause, and the thoughts and beliefs of your friends. It is a natural process, but it is a time of unpredictable swings in hormones and emotions. One month the estrogen levels may be high, the next month they may be low. Swings in hormones can cause difficulty sleeping, mood swings, and foggy thinking and can affect your blood glucose control.

The symptoms experienced during menopause can often be confused with the symptoms of low and even high blood glucose. Hot flashes, moodiness, and short-term memory loss can be mistaken as low blood glucose, when in fact they are related to shifts in hormone levels. It is important for you to check your blood glucose level before assuming that it is low and eating unnecessary calories. You may also see wide swings in glycemic control as the levels of hormones change or as a result of inadequate sleep.

During menopause, women often report low blood glucose levels that are stronger and more frequent, especially during the middle of the night. Sleep is often disrupted. Controlling your diabetes can be difficult—as it is for teenagers, who also experience wide swings in hormone levels. When the hormone levels increase, blood glucose increases as well. Dealing with the unpredictability of blood glucose and hot flashes can leave you feeling frustrated and sad.

Keep your diabetes regimen going, get adequate sleep, and try relaxation techniques to help balance the effects of emotional and physical stress. Nap when you need to, and learn to breathe!

As the levels of the hormones estrogen and progesterone decrease, your body will be less resistant to insulin.

Some women experience more hypoglycemia. You may find that you need to decrease the dose of your insulin or diabetes pills during or after menopause. Another body change that you may see during and after menopause is vaginal dryness, resulting in painful intercourse and increased risk for urinary tract infections. Persistent high blood glucose levels can make this condition worse. Cream and gel lubricants can be used during sexual activity. Prompt treatment of vaginal and urinary tract infections is important.

Hormone replacement therapy (HRT) is an option for some women. Good nutrition, weight training, aerobic exercise, and sleep are the foundation for a healthy transition during menopause. You may want to consider yoga, meditation, and other stress reduction techniques to help relieve the symptoms and enhance your overall feeling of well-being.

A dietitian can help review your needs for calcium supplements and make changes to your meal plan. Some women report that calcium-magnesium supplements help to reduce headaches, irritability, depression, and insomnia. Calcium can be found in high amounts in dairy products; green, leafy vegetables like broccoli; cauliflower; pinto beans and soybeans; and nuts such as brazil nuts, hazel nuts, and almonds. The daily requirement for calcium before menopause is 1,000 mg/day. Post-menopausal women need 1,000 mg if they are on HRT and 1,500 mg if they are not. Calcium replacement will also help prevent osteoporosis. Some women report success using a higher soy diet and supplementing with bioflavinoids. If you choose to supplement with herbs, be aware that herbs are like medicines and must be taken under the supervision of someone trained in this area.

If you are on HRT and start taking troglitazone (Rezulin) to control your diabetes, check with your physician to see if your estrogen doses need to be increased.

How does menopause affect your heart?

Estrogen provides a certain degree of protection against heart disease. Estrogen, released from the ovaries, helps to increase the production of HDL cholesterol, the good cholesterol, and to break down LDL cholesterol, the bad cholesterol. It also relaxes the smooth muscle of the blood vessels. Once a woman experiences menopause, the production of estrogen goes down.

As a woman with diabetes, you are at risk for developing heart disease earlier than your friends without diabetes. Diabetes negates the protective effects of estrogen and puts you at risk for heart disease and a life-threatening heart attack. If you have heart disease, discuss with your provider what your target blood glucose range should be. It is generally recommended to try to avoid hypoglycemia because of the increased chance of having a heart attack. (See chapter 5 about your heart.)

How do menopause and diabetes put you at risk for osteoporosis?

As a woman ages, her bones tend to become weaker, putting her at risk for osteoporosis. Yet there are things you can do today to protect your bones.

Osteoporosis, which means "porous bone," is a condition in which bone mass is lost as a result of losing minerals and protein. Bones become very fragile and fracture easily. Estrogen, calcium, vitamin D, and weight-bearing exercise are important to the health and strength of your bones. Even though all humans lose a little bone mass, not all women are at risk for osteoporosis. Some men develop it, too.

You are more at risk for osteoporosis if you are a smoker, thin, fair skinned, have experienced menopause early, have been on steroid therapy, or have had prolonged high blood glucose levels. In addition, if you do not take in enough calories or calcium, or you have a history of anorexia or bulimia, your bones have not received the nutrients they need to stay strong. If you have been caught up in quick-weight-loss diet fads or have a diet low in calcium, high in alcohol and caffeine, or very low in fat, your bones have probably been weakened. Your body needs a little bit of dietary fat to make estrogen, which is needed for building bone and preventing bone loss.

Because most women with type 2 diabetes are overweight, they are less likely to develop osteoporosis. However, this is not true if their blood glucose levels are always high. Exercise is the best way to increase muscle mass and protect your bones.

How is osteoporosis prevented and treated?

No matter what age you are, you should consider the suggestions below.

- Engage in weight-bearing exercise, which helps to increase body mass and density. Exercise should vary. Your body will respond nicely to exercise that involves repetition and muscle strengthening of the large muscle groups. Even lifting 1 or 2 pounds helps increase bone mass and muscle strength
- Stop smoking! Smoking interferes with calcium absorption and leaves the bone fragile and thin. Smoking is also a risk because smokers tend to eat

a high-fat diet, drink excess alcohol, and exercise less—all risk factors for developing osteoporosis.

- Eat a balanced meal plan that has enough calcium, phosphorus, and vitamin D. Ask a dietitian how you can increase these minerals in your diet.
- Get your diabetes under control!
- Consider HRT or other medications (Calcitonin, Fosamax), especially if you are at high risk or if you are postmenopausal. Explore this option and its side effects with your provider

Lois Jovanovic, MD; Mark A. Sperling, MD; Leslie R. Schover, PhD; Ilana P. Spector, PhD; Patricia Schreiner-Engel, PhD; and Laurinda M. Poirier, RN, MPH, CDE, contributed to this chapter.

19

Oral Health

Case study

PJ is a 19-year-old woman with type 1 diabetes. She has an abscessed (infected) wisdom tooth, and her dentist has recommended the removal of all four wisdom teeth. The oral surgeon, conferring with PJ's physician, may recommend a temporary reduction in insulin dosage after the extractions, because she won't be able to eat after the surgery. She will be closely monitored to prevent the development of diabetic ketoacidosis (chapter 1) or hypoglycemia (chapter 2).

Introduction

People with diabetes may develop a variety of oral problems, including gum disease and infections. Seemingly routine dental problems like gum infections and abscesses from bad teeth can have a significant impact on blood sugar levels, upsetting the fragile balance that you achieve with healthy eating and medication.

Toothaches, gum disease, or any oral condition that can interfere with your ability to eat takes on added significance. Because healthy eating is such a key element to your control of the disease, it is even more important to maintain a healthy mouth. The key to good oral health is to focus on preventive care through regular checkups and cleanings and an oral hygiene program at home.

How does diabetes affect your mouth and teeth?

Diabetes affects the mouth in three ways:

1. High blood glucose has an effect on the small blood vessels of the body. In the mouth it contributes to gum disease and slowed healing.

2. People with diabetes have difficulty fighting off infections in the mouth, for example, abscesses that come from deep cavities or gum disease. Their white blood cells show diminished capacity to fight off invading bacteria.

3. Diabetes can lead to an oral condition known as *xerostomia*, or dry mouth. This decrease in saliva production may be caused by autonomic neuropathy and can have several effects, including an increased incidence of cavities and oral fungal and bacterial infections.

What is periodontal disease?

Periodontal disease may be referred to as *gum disease, gingivitis*, or *periodontitis*. These are all terms referring to the breakdown of the structures that support the teeth—the gums and bone. Just as a poor foundation will ruin an otherwise sound building, healthy teeth are often lost because of periodontal disease.

In a healthy mouth, the roots of the teeth are solidly encased in bone, the *alveolus*. The soft tissue (the gums) covers the bone and wraps around each tooth up to the base of the crown (Figure 19-1). As a consequence of this configuration, a space exists around the tooth between it and the gums called the *periodontal pocket*. This is where a dental instrument, or toothbrush bristle, or dental floss goes when we say these things are "under the gumline."

Two types of material build up on the teeth above the gumline and below in the pocket: *plaque* and *calculus* (also called tartar). Plaque is a soft film that can be removed with normal brushing and flossing. Calculus is the harder material that is removed by dentists and dental hygienists during regular cleaning sessions. Both are rich in bacteria and cause irritation to the gums. If plaque and calculus are allowed to remain in contact with the teeth and gums, periodontal disease can develop and progress through several stages.

What are the symptoms of gum disease?

In gingivitis, the earliest stage of gum disease, the gums are red and swollen and bleed easily. After the thorough removal of all plaque and calculus, the gums will return to normal. If this material is not removed and the situation progresses, the gumline will begin to recede, exposing some of the root surface (Figure 19-2). As the gumline continues to move, the level of the bone starts to recede as well. Eventually, after enough bone has been lost, the teeth will loosen and will need to be extracted or may come out on their own (Figure 19-3). At any point in this progression, a thorough cleaning and the implementation of good oral home care will stop the gum recession and bone loss. However, the lost gum and underlying bone cannot be made to grow back.

What is the connection between periodontal disease and diabetes?

According to data from the National Health and Nutrition Examination Survey, Americans with diabetes are more than twice as likely as the general population to experience some form of gum disease. Clearly, you are at a significantly greater risk for periodontal disease because:

- The impact of diabetes on the small blood vessels of the gums creates a situation where the blood flow to the gum tissue is reduced; so the gums do not receive a good supply of the nutrients and oxygen normally supplied by the blood.
- The white blood cells responsible for fighting bacteria function poorly in people with diabetes. The plaque and calculus on the teeth and below the gumline are bacteria rich.
- A higher level of glucose in saliva may attract more destructive bacteria.
- People with diabetes have problems manufacturing collagen, a major building block of the gums.

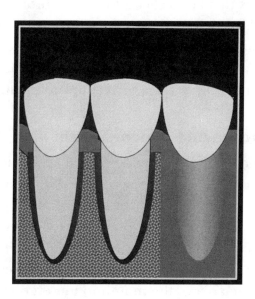

Figure 19-1. Anatomy of healthy teeth/gums/bone. Note the height of the bone and the tightness of the gums against the teeth.

Gum infections can, in turn, affect your diabetes. Infection can significantly raise your blood glucose levels and oral medication or insulin requirements.

How is gum disease diagnosed?

A thorough dental examination will turn up several indicators for the presence of periodontal disease.

1. Visual exam—red, swollen gums and the presence of visible plaque and calculus accumulated on the surface of the teeth and below the gumline
2. Radiographic (X-ray) exam—level of the bone that supports the teeth and any bone loss that has taken place
3. Periodontal charting—series of measurements including the depth of the pocket that surrounds each tooth

The teeth themselves must also be evaluated to identify areas that are difficult to clean—broken teeth and fillings; older, defective caps or crowns; rotated, misaligned teeth; and poorly fitting partial plates. Based on this examination, your dentist evaluates the state of health of your gums and decides on a course of treatment.

What is the treatment for gum disease?

Treatment for gum disease can be as simple as routine dental cleanings performed every 3–6 months. If the amounts of plaque and calculus are more significant and/or the periodontal pockets are deeper, your dentist may recommend another treatment, a scaling and root planing. This deep cleaning usually involves several visits where the area of the mouth to undergo treatment is numbed with local anesthetic. When the procedure is completed, you may need to return more frequently than every 6 months for check ups.

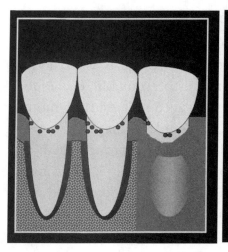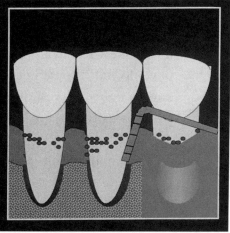

Figures 19-2 and 19-3. Moderate and advanced gum disease. Note the tartar build up and the destruction of bone. We would expect the teeth in figure 19-3 to be loose.

In more severe cases, the loss of bony support for the teeth is more extensive, and the depth of the periodontal pockets makes it difficult or impossible to perform a thorough cleaning. You may be referred to a dental specialist concerned with gum problems—the periodontist. The periodontist uses many techniques for returning the gums to a healthy state, some of which involve surgical procedures performed in the office on an outpatient basis. A major goal of periodontal surgery is to reshape the bone and reposition the gums to create an oral landscape that is easily cleaned and maintained. When periodontal pockets get deep enough, it becomes impossible to clean the entire space with a toothbrush and dental floss. The result is that material continues to accumulate in the pocket, causing further irritation and recession of the soft tissue and thus a deeper pocket. As the pocket deepens and the gumline recedes, the bone level recedes, making the teeth loose. This begins a cycle that, without intervention, can end in tooth loss.

How can you prevent gum disease?

Although it is true that people who have diabetes are more likely to have periodontal disease, it is also true that periodontal disease is completely preventable. If plaque and calculus are not allowed to accumulate in the mouth, your gums stay healthy. It is as simple as that.

Once you have seen a dentist for a thorough cleaning and the elimination of problem areas and plaque traps, it is essential to embark on a conscientious home-care program. For most people, this is just a matter of brushing after meals and flossing daily. There are many aids to oral hygiene available. For example, people with fixed bridge-work cannot clean between or under the teeth on a bridge with regular dental floss and so require some additional implement (of which there are several brands). Electric toothbrushes may be helpful for people who have trouble with regular brushing and flossing. The thing to remember is that every mouth is different, and different people get different results with different techniques. Critical is the development of a home-care routine suited to you. This may also include prescription products such as medicated rinses and toothpastes designed to kill bacteria and control bleeding and inflammation.

What other infections can occur in your mouth?

Severe dental disease can cause swings in blood glucose levels. This is true for gum disease as well as two other conditions: *thrush* and *xerostomia* (dry mouth).

What is thrush and how is it treated?

Candidiasis, or thrush, is a yeastlike fungal infection. It may appear in your mouth as white patches or as red areas of irritation. A sensation of soreness or burning sometimes accompanies this change in appearance, making dentures uncomfortable or impossible to wear. Candidiasis in people with diabetes may be the result of an increase in the amount of glucose in the saliva. The reduced flow of saliva often experienced by people with diabetes may also contribute to this.

This condition is treated with prescription medications that are available in several forms, including rinses, ointments, lozenges, and pills.

How does dry mouth affect your oral health?

Xerostomia, or dry mouth, is thought to be due to autonomic neuropathy. A lack of saliva is an annoyance in itself, making eating and speaking more difficult and causing a bad taste and odor. It can also make you more likely to get cavities in your teeth.

Saliva serves several distinct purposes—a digestive enzyme, a lubricant, and a self-cleaning element of the mouth. Salivation helps to minimize the amount of food debris that remains in contact with the teeth after eating. When your ability to salivate is impaired, you are likely to have a dramatic increase in the formation of cavities.

How is dry mouth treated?

To combat the effects of dry mouth, your dentist may prescribe fluoride gels or rinses to strengthen the teeth and remineralize (fill in) small cavities. These products have a higher fluoride content than over-the-counter toothpastes and should only be used with the advice of a dentist. Another prescription product is artificial saliva that can be sipped and swished to aid you in eating and speaking.

Some nonprescription techniques that are simple and effective involve gum, candy, cantaloupe juice, or water. Gum and hard candies (sugarless, of course) will stimulate the flow of saliva. Studies have conclusively shown that chewing sugarless gum after meals does decrease cavity formation. Increasing the amount of water that you drink will minimize dehydration. Constant sipping throughout the day and during meals will fulfill the role of the saliva in lubricating your mouth. Ice chips are good for this as well.

Will your diabetes interfere with dental treatment?

Before considering the possible problems involved in dental treatment for an individual with diabetes, a couple of distinctions must be made. The first is between a person with uncontrolled blood glucose levels and a person with well-controlled diabetes (closer-to-normal blood glucose levels). The next distinction is between routine and extensive dental treatment. Routine dental treatment requires minimal anesthesia, short appointments, and causes little or no bleeding. Procedures such as fillings and simple cleanings are in this category. More extensive procedures involve longer appointments and more local anesthetic and may cause more bleeding. This would include the extraction of several teeth, multiple crowns or bridges, or any surgical procedure.

People with well-controlled diabetes can undergo routine dental treatment the same as anyone else, although some general precautions should always be taken. Local anesthetic with epinephrine should be avoided on many people with diabetes, especially those who have had diabetes for a long time, because it causes a rapid heartbeat (tachycardia). You should ask your dentist about this.

People who take insulin or oral medications are best scheduled for midmorning appointments, after taking their medication and eating a normal breakfast. If you monitor your blood glucose, always inform your dentist of the most recent number. Always ask how long the "numbness" will last—your dentist can use shorter-acting anesthetics so that you do not have to skip or postpone a meal. Remember, eating while numb from local anesthetic can cause injury.

People with well-controlled diabetes can usually undergo more extensive dental procedures without problems, but it is important for you, your dentist, and your physician to determine if any special precautions need to be taken. Infection, pain, and stress can all affect your blood glucose levels.

People with uncontrolled blood glucose pose a more challenging case for dental care. Because of frequent fluctuations in your blood glucose levels, your dentist and physician must consult even for your routine dental treatment. For people with diabetes who are unaware of the status of their disease and who are not under the regular care of a physician, only minimal procedures are performed to relieve pain in emergency situations until their overall health can be assessed (Figure 19-4).

If you have heart valve disease, you may need protective doses of antibiotics. Always report any heart problems to your dentist. Dental treatment should begin with a thorough medical history and close communication between you, your dentist, and your physician.

What should you consider when scheduling a dental appointment?

Another point to consider is how to manage your dental appointment to minimize your chances of hypoglycemia, or low blood glucose levels. Never skip a meal or a dose of medication before or after a dental appointment unless you are told to do so by your physician. If you're not sure, check with your diabetes team. Dental treatment can cause people to feel anxious, but it is important to keep stress to a minimum. Stress and anxiety can bring on hyperglycemia in some people. Some people may need sedation with nitrous oxide ("laughing gas"). Your dentist may choose to prescribe an anti-anxiety medication to be taken the night before and on the morning of the dental visit. Most people only need the numbing action of the local anesthetic to be comfortable throughout the dental procedure.

What happens after your dental treatment?

After dental treatment, find out how long you can expect to be numb and whether there will be any discomfort as the numbness wears off. These two factors affect your ability to eat and so to maintain a consistent blood glucose level. You may need to switch to a soft or liquid diet temporarily, or in extreme cases, the dosage of your medication may need to be reduced. Consult with your physician before you do this. Also, for some patients with diabetes, healing time may be longer and the risk of infection may be greater. Therefore, depending on the nature of the work performed, your dentist may ask to see you for a follow-up visit or may need to prescribe an antibiotic.

In conclusion

Diabetes can cause problems in the mouth, and problems in the mouth can create difficulties in managing diabetes. Preventive care is a powerful weapon from either perspective: People with well-controlled diabetes are unlikely to experience the oral problems associated with diabetes, and people who take good care of their mouths are unlikely to have dental problems severe enough to affect their diabetes.

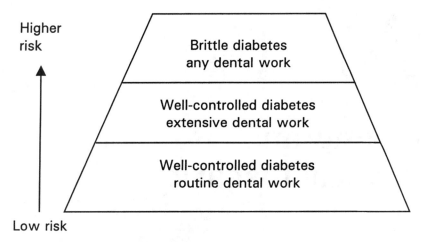

Higher risk

Brittle diabetes
any dental work

Well-controlled diabetes
extensive dental work

Well-controlled diabetes
routine dental work

Low risk

Figure 19-4. Diabetes and dental treatment—pyramid of risk.

Dental treatment may be more complicated for people with diabetes, but it depends on the status of their disease and the specific procedure being performed. Dental treatments can be managed in a straightforward manner as long as there is good communication between your dentist, your physician, and you.

This chapter was written by Jeffrey A. Levin, DMD.

20

Obesity and Physical Inactivity

Case study

DS and HA are Pima Indians. They are distant cousins. DS lives in the U.S. and works for a construction company. HA lives in Mexico, where he and his family farm for a living. Like most of his neighbors, DS eats a lot of high-fat and sugary foods. He has a sedentary lifestyle when he's not at work. Like his neighbors, HA eats a lot of foods high in complex carbohydrates, such as beans and corn tortillas. Farming keeps him constantly active. DS has had type 2 diabetes for 5 years. HA has normal blood glucose levels.

Introduction

Obesity and physical inactivity are not complications of diabetes, rather diabetes can be seen as a complication of obesity and physical inactivity. This chapter discusses the link between obesity and physical activity and their effect on both the risk of developing diabetes and the management of it. In addition, because diabetes is associated with an increased risk of coronary heart disease (CHD), this chapter also briefly discusses the importance of weight and activity in preventing CHD. (See chapter 5 for more on heart disease.)

Obesity and physical inactivity are associated with the development of type 2 diabetes. In fact, 80% of people with type 2 diabetes are overweight. In contrast, most people with type 1 diabetes are normal weight. Thus, the focus of this chapter is on people with type 2 diabetes.

Why do some people get diabetes and some not?

Both genetics and environment contribute to the development of type 2 diabetes (Figure 20-1). If one of your parents, siblings, or grandparents has diabetes, you are at increased risk of developing the disease. However, your behavior has a big influence on whether you develop this disease. People who are overweight and/or inactive are at increased risk of developing diabetes. Even if you have a strong genetic background for diabetes, maintaining a healthy body weight and an active lifestyle can help prevent the occurrence of diabetes.

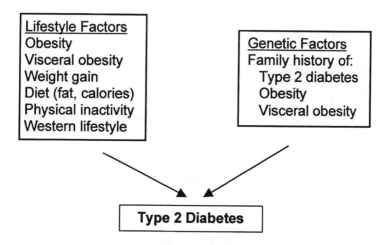

Figure 20-1. Interactions between lifestyle and genetics that can lead to type 2 diabetes.

A recent study illustrates this point very well. The Pima Indians who live in Arizona have the highest rates of diabetes of any group in the U.S.—75% of the adults have it. They clearly have a strong genetic predisposition to develop this disease. The Arizona Pimas live a Westernized lifestyle—they eat high-fat foods, get very little exercise, and are overweight. The combination of a strong genetic predisposition and high obesity, high-fat foods, and low activity unfortunately makes diabetes extremely common in this population.

In contrast, another group of Pima Indians, who live in a rural area of Mexico, appear to have very low rates of diabetes. The Mexican Pimas, by all evidence, have the same genetic background as the Arizona Pimas and thus are apparently at high risk of developing the disease. However, the Pimas in Mexico still live a farming lifestyle, with high levels of physical activity (for example, farming the fields without modern tools) and a diet high in complex carbohydrates. The Mexican Pimas have low rates of obesity and low rates of diabetes. Despite a common genetic background, the differences in activity and diet of the two groups create significant differences in how many of them get diabetes.

How do obesity and physical activity increase the risk of diabetes?

People who are genetically predisposed to diabetes and obesity may have abnormalities in the amount of insulin they produce and/or in their ability to use the insulin that their pancreas produces. Inactivity and obesity also make the body less able to use the insulin it produces (referred to as insulin resistance). For a while, the pancreas is able to overcome insulin resistance by increasing the amount of insulin it produces (hyperinsulinemia), and blood glucose remains normal. However, over time, the ability of the pancreas to produce these higher levels of insulin decreases; if the pancreas cannot continue to make enough insulin to overcome the insulin resistance, blood glucose levels rise, and diabetes develops. Increased physical activity and weight loss can improve how the body uses the insulin it does make and prevent this sequence from occurring.

What levels of body weight are associated with diabetes?

The chance of developing diabetes is increased when you are very overweight. However, it is unclear what level of body weight is ideal—that is, the weight that has the lowest risk of being associated with diabetes. Several factors may influence this, including the way the body weight is distributed and the amount of weight you have gained over your life.

In the past, obesity was based on a comparison to an "ideal body weight," which is difficult to define. Today, it is more common to use the body mass index (BMI), which corrects body weight for height (Table 20-1).

In most healthy individuals, a BMI above 27 is considered obese. This cutoff level is based on several large studies that showed a greater chance of early death when the BMI was above this level. Although this cutoff applies to most people, it does not apply to well-trained athletes, who may have a higher BMI because of high levels of muscle mass, or to pregnant women.

A BMI of 27 may be too high if you already have medical conditions that are known to be associated with obesity. These medical conditions include type 2 diabetes, high blood pressure, and high cholesterol. For people with these health problems or a strong family history of these diseases, a BMI of less than 25 is recommended. Some studies have suggested that the lowest risk of developing diabetes occurs at a BMI of approximately 21.

In addition to the total amount of fat, where the body fat is located is also important. An increased amount of fat in the abdomen (apple shape) is more strongly associated with diabetes than is body fat on the hips (pear shape) (Figure 20-1). Abdominal obesity is also associated with hypertension, hyperlipidemia (high triglycerides and low levels of HDL cholesterol, the "good" cholesterol) and CHD.

Several factors influence the distribution of body fat. One is sex—men have more abdominal fat than women. A second is your genetic background—parents and children often resemble each other in fat patterning. Finally, several behavioral factors increase abdominal obesity, including low physical activity, smoking, stress, and eating a lot of high-fat foods.

The best way to determine whether you have abdominal obesity without expensive procedures is to measure your waist. A waist circumference of more than 35 inches in women or 40 inches in men suggests this is the case.

Studies have shown that weight gain since age 18 is another important factor in determining the risk of diabetes. Individuals who have gained more than 20 pounds since age 18 are at increased risk of developing diabetes. This is of particular concern because it is so common for individuals to gain weight as they age.

How does what you eat increase your risk of diabetes?

Eating too much sugar is not the problem; there is little evidence that high sugar intake is the cause of diabetes. Most studies suggest that it is the amount of fat in the

Table 20.1 Body Mass Index (BMI) Values

BMI

Height	19	20	21	22	23	24	25	26	27	28	29	30	31	32	33	34	35	36	37	38	39	40
	Good Weights									Weight (in pounds)						Increasing Risk						
4'10"	91	96	100	105	110	115	119	124	129	134	138	143	148	153	158	162	167	172	177	181	186	191
4'11"	94	99	104	109	114	119	124	128	133	138	143	148	153	158	163	168	173	178	183	188	193	198
5'	97	102	107	112	118	123	128	133	138	143	148	153	158	163	168	174	179	184	189	194	199	204
5'1"	100	106	111	116	122	127	132	137	143	148	153	158	164	169	174	180	185	190	195	201	206	211
5'2"	104	109	115	120	126	131	136	142	147	153	158	164	169	175	180	186	191	196	202	207	213	218
5'3"	107	113	118	124	130	135	141	146	152	158	163	169	175	180	186	191	197	203	208	214	220	225
5'4"	110	116	122	128	134	140	145	151	157	163	169	174	180	186	192	197	204	209	215	221	227	232
5'5"	114	120	126	132	138	144	150	156	162	168	174	180	186	192	198	204	210	216	222	228	234	240
5'6"	118	124	130	136	142	148	155	161	167	173	179	186	192	198	204	210	216	223	229	235	241	247
5'7"	121	127	134	140	146	153	159	166	172	178	185	191	198	204	211	217	223	230	236	242	249	255
5'8"	125	131	138	144	151	158	164	171	177	184	190	197	203	210	216	223	230	236	243	249	256	262
5'9"	128	135	142	149	155	162	169	176	182	189	196	203	209	216	223	230	236	243	250	257	263	270
5'10"	132	139	146	153	160	167	174	181	188	195	202	209	216	222	229	236	243	250	257	264	271	278
5'11"	136	143	150	157	165	172	179	186	193	200	208	215	222	229	236	243	250	257	265	272	279	286
6'	140	147	154	162	169	177	184	191	199	206	213	221	228	235	242	250	258	265	272	279	287	294
6'1"	144	151	159	166	174	182	189	197	204	212	219	227	235	242	250	257	265	272	280	288	295	302
6'2"	148	155	163	171	179	186	194	202	210	218	225	233	241	249	256	264	272	280	288	295	303	311
6'3"	152	160	168	176	184	192	200	208	216	224	232	240	248	256	264	272	279	287	295	303	311	319
6'4"	156	164	172	180	189	197	205	213	221	230	238	246	254	263	271	279	287	295	304	312	320	328

BMI ≥27 are highlighted because health risk escalates rapidly above this level.

diet, rather than the amount of carbohydrate, that increases the risk of diabetes. You should be aware of the amount of fat you are eating for several reasons. First, fat is fattening. Each gram of fat you eat (a gram is about the weight of a paper clip) provides 9 calories. In contrast, each gram of carbohydrate (fruits, grains, vegetables) has 4 calories and each gram of protein (in meats, fish, poultry, milk) has 4 calories. Gram for gram, fat is twice as fattening as carbohydrates or protein. Dietary fats, especially saturated fat, can also raise your cholesterol levels. Because people with diabetes are at increased risk of heart disease, it is important to watch dietary fat intake to reduce the risk of CHD.

You should see a dietitian for help determining your target levels for fat and protein and carbohydrate. Your meal plan should be developed to suit your needs and goals.

What is the relationship between physical activity and diabetes?

Many studies show the strong effect of physical activity on the chances of developing diabetes. In these studies, a large group of middle-aged people are examined initially when they do not have diabetes. They are followed to see who will develop diabetes. In the Nurses Health Study, more than 80,000 nurses aged 35–59 were followed for 8 years. Women who engaged in vigorous activity at least one time per week had a lower risk of developing diabetes than those who were less active. In fact, the major difference was between the women who reported no physical activity and those who exercised at least one time per week.

Being inactive increases the chance that you will be overweight, and overweight increases your risk of dia-

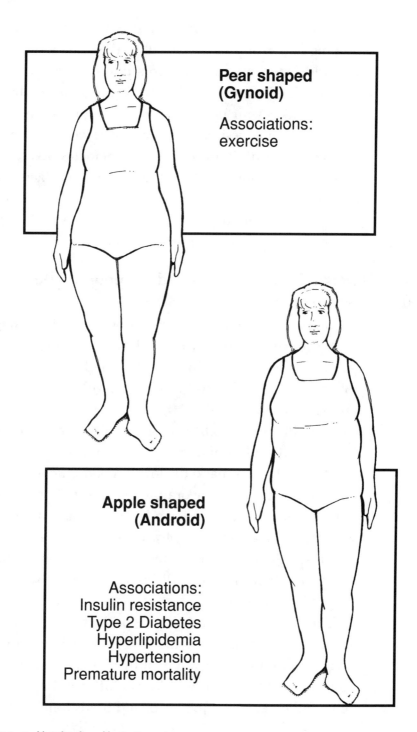

Pear shaped (Gynoid)

Associations:
exercise

Apple shaped (Android)

Associations:
Insulin resistance
Type 2 Diabetes
Hyperlipidemia
Hypertension
Premature mortality

Figure 20-1. Health Risk Indicated by Fat Patterning.

betes. However, even if you adjust for this (for example, looking at a group of people all of the same weight), you will find that those people who are most active have the lowest risk of diabetes. This is probably because physical activity makes your body more sensitive to insulin (reduces insulin resistance), thereby decreasing the chance that you will develop type 2 diabetes. Exercise also helps reduce abdominal obesity, another risk factor for diabetes. Also important is the fact that increased physical activity lowers blood pressure levels and raises HDL cholesterol, giving you some protection against CHD.

Why is weight loss recommended for people with type 2 diabetes who are obese?

In the past, the goal of weight loss was to reduce weight to the "normal" range. We now know that weight losses of just 10–20 pounds can improve blood glucose, blood pressure, and cholesterol in patients with type 2 diabetes and reduce the risks of CHD.

The effects of weight loss on blood sugar control occur very quickly and dramatically. Just 1 or 2 weeks of lower calorie intake can markedly lower blood glucose levels. If you are using insulin or oral medication to control your diabetes notify your physician before embarking on a weight-loss program. The physician may want to adjust the dose of insulin or diabetes pills that you are taking and your hypertension medication before the start of the weight-loss program.

The only way to maintain the positive benefits of weight loss is to maintain the new body weight. This means continuing to eat a healthy diet and to exercise. If you lose 10–20 pounds and keep it off, you improve your blood glucose, blood pressure, and lipids long term.

What is the treatment for obesity?

The primary treatment for obesity is lifestyle change, involving change in both food choices and physical activity. Many people find it helpful to have the support of a group in making these changes (for example, TOPS, Overeaters Anonymous, or your diabetes support group).

The most effective lifestyle changes for the treatment of obesity include changing what you eat, increasing your physical activity, learning behavior modification, and getting ongoing support from a health care provider. The following suggestions may be helpful:

1. To lose weight, you need to change energy balance—the amount of energy (calories) you take in through eating and the amount of energy you use up through exercise. The most effective approach to long-term weight loss is to change both sides of the energy-balance equation: eat less and exercise more.

2. To get an idea of what you are currently eating, write down everything you eat for 1 week. Be careful to write down *everything*, and be precise about describing the food and the serving size. Use a calorie and fat guide or the food label to figure out how many calories and grams of fat you are eating.

3. To lose weight, you need to eat less than you are currently eating. To lose 1–2 pounds per week, which is considered the best rate of weight loss, you need to reduce the amount of calories you are eating by 500–1,000 calories per day. If you find that you usually eat 2,000 calories, you should eat 1,100–1,500 calories/day to lose weight. Do not go below 1,000 calories per day or you run the risk of getting sick. To get as much

food as possible at a calorie level, consider your fat intake. Remember, fat has more than twice as many calories per gram as protein or carbohydrate. Write down what you ea,t and figure out the calories and fat grams you are consuming. Writing down what you eat helps you track your progress over time. You may need to see a registered dietitian (RD) for help developing a balanced meal plan for you.

4. Increase your physical activity in the form of brisk walking. Check with your physician before embarking on any physical activity more vigorous than walking. Start slowly and build up gradually to avoid injury. Any physical activity burns calories. You don't need to jog a mile to burn calories; walking the mile works just as well. You don't need to go out and exercise for 40 minutes to burn calories; four short walks of 10 minutes each will do just as well! Gradually increase your daily activity until you are walking for 30 minutes each day or about 2 miles a day.

5. Set up your home to support your healthier lifestyle. It is easier to follow an eating plan if you buy healthy foods and have them available. Don't purchase high-fat snack items such as chips, crackers, nuts, or cheese. The principle is: "Out of sight is out of mind." Do the reverse for physical activity. If you own an exercise bike, put it where you see it so it reminds you to exercise. Keep your walking shoes close by.

6. Set a goal of losing 10–20 pounds and keeping it off. Modest weight losses of 10–20 pounds are effective in reducing the risk of obesity-related health problems and help to treat those problems.

The Uncomplicated Guide to Diabetes Complications

Are there medications for the treatment of obesity?

Several medications are currently available for the treatment of obesity. These medications promote weight loss by decreasing your appetite or increasing your feeling of fullness. However, to work, they must be used with changes in diet and physical activity.

Weight losses with prescription medication have averaged 5–20 pounds higher than those seen with nondrug treatments, but the maximum weight loss typically occurs at 6 months, followed by a plateau in weight or weight regain.

Appetite suppressants are recommended primarily for people who are significantly obese or have health problems associated with their obesity. These medications, like all medications, have side effects. Most of the side effects are mild, although rare, serious and even fatal outcomes have been reported. Appetite-suppressant medications should **not** be used by someone who wants to lose just a few pounds. Consult your physician.

How can I learn more about weight and physical activity?

There is a tremendous amount of misinformation available about obesity and physical activity. Useful and accurate information can be obtained from the Weight-Control Information Network (WIN). WIN is a service of the National Institute of Diabetes and Digestive and Kidney Diseases, a division of the National Institutes of Health. They can be contacted at:

Weight-Control Information Network
1 Win Way, Bethesda, MD 20892-3665
Phone: (800) 946-8098, Fax (301)570-2186

This chapter was written by Rena R. Wing, PhD, and Katherine V. Williams, MD.

The Uncomplicated Guide to Diabetes Complications

Appendix A: Screening to Prevent Complications

Complication	What to do
Eyes	Yearly dilated eye exam by eye specialist who is familiar with diabetes complications and treatment.
Kidneys	Yearly microalbumin and clearance test
Nerves	Yearly check with monofilaments
Cholesterol	LDL < 100
Blood pressure	< 140/85
Glycosylated hemoglobin	Every 3 months
Feet	Check for neuropathy and foot deformity at least twice a year.

Appendix B: Diabetes Prevention Program

The federally funded Diabetes Prevention Program (DPP) is to determine whether progression from impaired glucose tolerance (IGT) to diabetes can be prevented or slowed down by lifestyle changes or medications.

The goal of DPP is to recruit approximately 50% of study volunteers from the African American, Hispanic, Asian, Pacific Islander, and American Indian communities. Within each ethnic group, participants are selected based on their high risk for future development of diabetes. This risk is determined by a screening process that utilizes information on height, weight, family history of diabetes, history of gestational diabetes, and blood glucose levels, among others. There are 25 DPP centers nationwide; most centers will continue recruiting volunteers through the year 2000, and the study is expected to close out by 2003. Call toll free at 1-888-377-5646 for more information.

The DPP is a good opportunity for family members of diabetes patients to enroll in a prevention trial. DPP also is an especially unique opportunity for people of ethnic heritage to participate in a clinical research program whose outcome can have an immense impact on the way the problem of diabetes is approached in the near future.

Glossary

albuminuria: the presence of protein in urine, usually a sign of disease, sometimes only temporary

androgen: a hormone that develops and maintains masculine characteristics

angina: a heart pain or pressure in the chest that may move to the arm, shoulder, or jaw

angioplasty: a surgical procedure done to open a blood vessel mechanically

angiotensin-converting enzyme (ACE) inhibitors: a class of drugs used to lower blood pressure and slow the progression of kidney disease

anticoagulants: blood thinners that help prevent formation of clots

antigens: foreign substances that trigger an immune response in your body

antibodies: part of your immune system, these are highly specific proteins called immunoglobulins that are produced by specialized cells in your body; they help the body identify and destroy antigens

arteriogram: an X ray using radioactive dye to view blood vessels

arteriole: the smallest blood vessel that has a wall

ascites: swelling caused by water accumulating in the tissues of the abdomen

asymptomatic: not having any symptoms

atherosclerosis: the process of cholesterol building up on the blood vessel walls, narrowing and sometimes blocking blood flow through them

autonomic neuropathy: damage to the nerves involved in involuntary processes such as heart beat or sweating *bacteriuria:* a urinary tract infection

brittle diabetes: an ongoing state of sharply fluctuating blood glucose levels that are difficult to control

CAD: coronary artery disease, in which some of the heart muscle does not receive sufficient blood, oxygen, and nutrients because of blockage of major blood vessels

cardiac catheterization: a procedure allowing examination of the blood vessels to the heart and the functioning of the different chambers of the heart

cardiac revascularization: repair or bypass of blocked blood vessels to the heart to restore circulation to the heart

cardioembolism: a blood clot in the arteries to the heart

cardiomyopathy: disease of the heart muscle

CDE: certified diabetes educator

cell-mediated immunity: the immune system defense by white blood cells that attack an antigen directly

cellulitis: a type of infection appearing as a red and tender swelling often on the feet or legs but also elsewhere

CHD: coronary heart disease, a disease of the blood vessels supplying the heart

CHF: congestive heart failure

cortisol: a counterregulatory or stress hormone that raises blood glucose levels

counterregulatory: a reaction that occurs to balance another process in the body

creatinine clearance: a test of kidney function that will show if an abnormally high amount of blood is passing through the kidney filters

CT (CAT): computed tomography, a special form of X-ray examination that quickly images an organ

cystitis: a urinary tract infection

DCCT: the Diabetes Control and Complications Trial, a 10-year study of the effects of tight control of blood glucose levels on complications in people with type 1 diabetes

dyspareunia: genital pain that occurs during or after intercourse when there is inadequate lubrication

DKA: diabetic ketoacidosis, a state of incomplete burning or metabolism of food causing high levels of acid in the blood that can lead to coma and sometimes death

dyslipidemia: high cholesterol and triglycerides, puts you at risk of atherosclerosis

edema: swelling caused by fluid building up in tissues of the body

ECG: electrocardiogram, a test to check for abnormal cardiac rhythm *echocardiogram:* an ultrasound test to check an organ for blood clots or other abnormalities

epinephrine: also known as adrenaline, a counterregulatory or stress hormone that raises blood glucose levels

ESRD: end-stage renal disease, damage to the kidneys so great that either dialysis or a transplant is necessary

essential hypertension: high blood pressure for which no cause is found

focal laser treatment: laser surgery, also called photocoagulation, to the retina of the eye

fructose: a sugar that occurs naturally in fruit and honey

gastroparesis: stomach paralysis

gastroesophageal reflux: heartburn

genitourinary: having to do with the genitals and urinary tract

gestational diabetes: diabetes that develops only during pregnancy

glomerulus: a complex of tiny blood vessel loops in the individual nephrons in a kidney that help filter the blood

glucagon: a hormone that raises blood glucose levels

glycated hemoglobin: (HbA_{1c}) a test to measure blood glucose levels over 2–3 months

growth hormone: a hormone that raises blood glucose levels

HDL cholesterol: high-density lipoproteins are fats made by the liver that collect excess cholesterol from the blood and blood vessels and transport it back to the liver, called the "good" cholesterol

hematologic: having to do with the components of the blood

HHNC: hyperglycemic hyperosmolar nonketotic coma, a dangerous state of extremely high blood glucose levels leading to coma and sometimes death

HRT: hormone replacement therapy for women during and after menopause to prevent osteoporosis, menopause symptoms, and heart disease

humoral immunity: the immune system defense that uses antibodies made by white blood cells called B-cells to ward off bacteria and viruses

hyperlipidemia: high levels of cholesterol and other fats in the blood

hypertension: high blood pressure

hypoglycemia unawareness: the loss or lack of any symptoms of hypoglycemia, sometimes because of nerve damage caused by diabetes

IGT: impaired glucose tolerance, occurs when the body cannot use some of the insulin that it makes, letting blood glucose levels run higher than normal but not in the diabetic
range

infarction: a sudden drop in blood supply to an organ or
area due to blood clots, twisting, or pressure (example: a
myocardial infarction is a heart attack)

insulin resistance: the body cannot efficiently use the
insulin that it produces

ischemia: poor blood circulation

ischemic stroke: a type of stroke caused by a lack of blood
supply to an area of the brain

IV: intravenous, usually refers to medication and nourishment
supplied to the body through a needle placed in a vein

IVP: intravenous pylogram, a special X-ray study using dye to
evaluate the structure of the kidneys

ketoacidosis (DKA): a state of incomplete burning or
metabolism of food causing a high level of acid in the blood
that can lead to coma

LDL cholesterol: low-density lipoproteins have a very high
concentration of cholesterol and are responsible for the
buildup in the walls of arteries that leads to atherosclerosis,
called the "bad" cholesterol

leukocytes: white blood cells

libido: sex drive

lymphocytes: a class of white blood cells that are responsible
for generating the body's immune response

macula: the center of the retina

macular edema: accumulation of fluid and swelling in the
macular area of the retina

magnetic resonance imaging (MRI): a test that uses a
large magnetic field and radio waves to produce a 3-dimen-
sional image of an organ without the use of any radiation

magnetic resonance angioscopy (MRA): a test that
examines the condition of blood vessels with a magnetic
field and radio waves instead of radiation or dyes

metatarsal: the long bones of the foot connecting toes and
ankle

microorganisms: an organism, such as a bacteria, visible
through a microscope

necrosis: breakdown or death of tissue

neovascularization: the growth of too many new blood
vessels that are fragile and easily leak

nephropathy: kidney or renal disease

nephrons: the 600,000 to 2 million subunits that make up the kidney filters

nephrotic syndrome: the changes that take place to damage the filters in the kidneys resulting in protein in the urine in quantities of 3,500 mg/day or more that is measurable by a dipstick test

neurogenic bladder: a bladder that cannot empty urine normally, perhaps because of nerve damage from diabetes

neuropathy: disease of the nerves

neutropenia: a reduction in the number of infection-fighting white blood cells in the body

noninvasive: a procedure that does not enter the body, not surgical

nonproliferative retinopathy: diabetic retinopathy marked by pinpoint leaks in blood vessels to the retina and changes to the blood vessels

normal flora: the bacteria that normally grow on the body

NSAIDs: nonsteroidal anti-inflammatory drugs

orthostatic hypotension: a sudden drop in blood pressure caused by standing up from a seated position; can cause dizziness, lightheadedness, seeing black spots, or passing out

orthotic: a specially made form to put in the shoes to make them fit better or to support the foot and prevent an ulcer from forming

osteomyelitis: an infection in the bone

panretinal photocoagulation: laser surgery to the retina of the eye, used to treat diabetic retinopathy

pathogens: organisms that cause an infection

pericardial effusion: water building up in the tissues around the heart

peripheral vascular disease (PVD): a condition of plaque buildup narrowing arteries to the legs and limiting circulation

pleural effusion: water building up in tissues in the chest

proliferative retinopathy: a severe form of diabetic retinopathy that includes the growth of fragile, new blood vessels on the retina of the eye

proteinuria: protein appearing in the urine in amounts large enough to be measured by a dipstick test (3,500 mg/day or more), an indication of advancing kidney disease

pyelonephritis: an infection in the urinary tract

RD: registered dietitian

renovascular hypertension: high blood pressure within the kidneys caused by cholesterol narrowing the arteries to the kidneys *retinopathy:* disease of the retina of the eye

scatter laser photocoagulation: laser surgery for proliferative diabetic retinopathy involving approximately 1,800
laser applications to the retina

sensorimotor neuropathy: damage to the nerves of the
feet and hands particularly caused by long-term high levels
of blood glucose

sonogram: an examination of the inner tissues and structures
of the body by use of sound waves

sorbitol: a sugar alcohol

sphincter: a ringlike muscle that normally closes a bodily
passage or orifice and opens when the natural bodily
process triggers it

statins: a group of drugs used to lower LDL cholesterol

stent: a tiny metal device shaped like a spring or mesh cylinder, used to hold a blood vessel open after angioplasty

sudomotor: sweat glands

TENS: Transcutaneous Nerve Stimulation unit that blocks
pain in a limb by sending electrical impulses

testosterone: a male hormone

TIA: transient ischemic attack, a temporary physical event
such as sudden weakness or numbness of the face, arm, or
leg that warns of a possible stroke

TPA: tissue plasminogen activator, a therapy for stroke that
dissolves clots, used within 3 hours after stroke symptoms
begin

triglycerides: fats that are carried in the blood but mostly
stored in fat tissue

tubule: a long path in the nephron of a kidney where urine
is filtered out and discharged into the bladder

UNOS: United Network for Organ Sharing, helps people find
and place donated organs such as kidneys

uremia: Greek word for urine in the blood

ureters: the duct or tubes carrying urine from the kidney to
the bladder

UTI: urinary tract infection

vaginismus: involuntary contractions of the vagina preventing penetration

vascular: having to do with the heart and blood vessels

Index